IT'S A POWERFUL LIFE

A GUIDE TO EVERYDAY FULFILLMENT THROUGH TRADITIONAL MARTIAL ARTS

By

Shifu Ahles

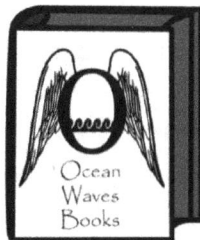

Ocean
Waves
Books

ISBN-10: 0-9989960-3-3

ISBN-13: 978-0-9989960-3-5

DISCLAIMER

The ideas expressed in this book are the opinion of the author unless otherwise indicated. The author can only offer his perspective of traditional martial arts practice and its philosophical teachings based on his own personal experience. The author expressly encourages you, the reader, to take it all with a grain of salt, make decisions for your life based on your own experiences, and ultimately trust your own inner guidance.

The information in this book is also meant to supplement, not replace, proper martial arts training. The application of any information contained in this book toward any endeavor is at the sole discretion of the reader.

Like any discipline involving speed, equipment, balance and environmental factors, martial arts and self defense training poses some inherent risk. The author advises readers to take full responsibility for their safety and know their limits. Before practicing anything described in this book, do not take risks beyond your level of experience, aptitude, training, and comfort level.

Dedication

To my wife, Nicolle, for all the years of unconditional love and never-ending support. I couldn't have done it without you.

Read This First!

Go to www.shifuahles.com/its-a-powerful-life

and claim your FREE GIFT!

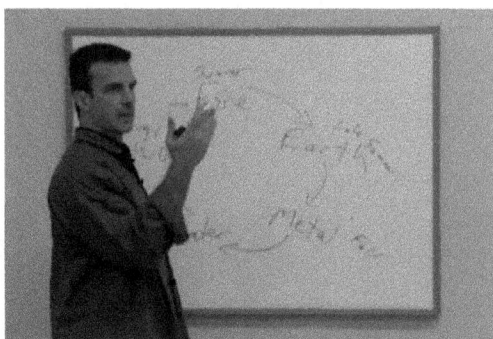

You have a FREE MEMBERSHIP waiting for you where you'll have access to many inspirational talks, recorded LIVE at our weekly meditation classes, that go above and beyond the topics covered in this book. If you like this book, you'll love these talks!

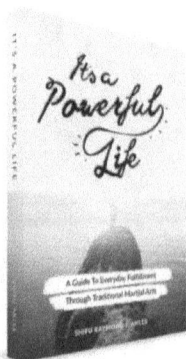

Table of Contents

A Wake-Up Call

My hope for this book is that it serves to inspire more people to do what is necessary to live a happy and fulfilling life. I have found the practice of traditional martial arts to be life-changing not only for me but also for the thousands of students I've worked with over the last thirty-plus years.

This practice is not an easy pursuit. The thing that is most satisfying for me is to watch a life change because they decide to do what they must.

If you're the kind of person who is willing to step up and do what it takes to overcome any self-imposed limiting beliefs you have so you can find success in your life one way or another, then this book, and traditional martial arts, are for you.

Your life will be better because of it.

Students of this practice learn first-hand that they can achieve any skill they choose, be it music, medicine, writing, or sport, as long as they are willing to put in the necessary consistent "effort over time," or, *Kung Fu*.

Kung, (gong, 功) literally translates as, "work, or effort."

The character *Fu,* (夫), literally means "adulthood, or grownup," inferring maturity, which takes "time."

I like to elaborate and expand on the meaning for clarity with, "achievement (or acquired skill) through consistent effort over time." This reveals how the term shines the light on both the journey and the destination.

When I use the term throughout this book, that is what is meant.

To be clear, any skill, in any endeavor, that a person has worked hard to acquire is Kung Fu. The term does not refer only to Chinese martial arts. A great doctor, dancer, gymnast, musician, or carpenter (and many others) would fit as well. *Think of anything where the great ones have acquired their knowledge and skills through consistent effort over time.*

Even the most successful salespeople or network marketers have to acquire their people skills, closing techniques, and the ability to remain calm while facing adversity (i.e. being unfazed by all the "No's" one must go through to get to a "Yes") through their consistent effort over time. And these teachings can help.

Of note here is that although I am generally consistent with my Romanization of Chinese words by using the modern standard known as *"Pinyin,"* I choose the more widely recognized *"Kung Fu"* versus the correct Pinyin *"Gong Fu"* throughout the book.

That said, I would also like to be clear and say that although my background is in the traditional Chinese martial arts, and I will often refer to the art and principles of one specific style known as, *"Ba Gua Zhang,"* as I know it, I do believe that what I am sharing here applies to all traditional martial arts of the East, which share a common philosophy.

In fact, I believe this philosophy and the concepts shared here can benefit people from all walks of life.

Now, let's start at the beginning...

Introduction

It was 1975, and I was 9 years of age when my new next door neighbor moved in. He was the same age, and I soon discovered he had been training in a tough inner city karate dojo for a few years.

As I got to know him, every once in a while, he'd show off some of his skills, one of which was "breaking." He once asked me to hold a broom stick in my hands as he proceeded to chop right through it with one swipe.

"Did that hurt?" I asked, which seemed like a logical question at the time.

"No." He responded, showing me how tough the knife-edge of his hand was from the conditioning they did at the dojo. I was impressed, and other kids who learned of his training sure didn't mess with him.

Just a few houses down the street lived a tough kid who was about a year older than me. He ran with the wrong crowd, and he always seemed to be in some sort of trouble. He'd frequently come storming out of his house yelling and cursing away at his parents. Then he'd usually make light of it if he happened to run into me on the way out.

But one time in the Spring of 1976, he didn't.

I was ten years old, out alone on the front lawn of my family's house minding my own business when I saw him walking by in the street.

I said, "Hi."

He murmured something as he walked over to me and punched me in the face. He followed up with a barrage of repeated punches to my left eye. I was on the ground, completely caught off guard by this and having no idea what to do.

All I could do to defend myself was grab hold of his shirt and tear it practically off him. This was clearly not a very effective response at all.

My parents were able to stop it before I was able to tear that shirt any further. Lucky for him! (ha, ha)

Well, the results were that my left eye was virtually swollen shut (think of the original "Rocky" movie) and I had to go to school where my classmates were sure to mock me. It was a humiliating experience, to say the least.

Defining Moments in our Lives

On that day, I was in the wrong place at the wrong time... *or was I?*

Something bad had happened to my neighbor, and there I was, in a convenient place for him to let out all that anger.

I swore revenge. I swore I would never be in that situation again. I would learn karate (the only martial arts term I knew back then), and I would get him back. I wanted that feeling of control so bad I could taste it. And I begged my parents to take me to a school.

They did, but I never took a lesson. I'm not sure what happened there.

Dad Takes Over

Growing up, I had heard stories about my father being a pretty tough kid as an adolescent in Jersey City in the 1940's and 50's. Neighborhood kids would get together and have bare-knuckled boxing matches in vacant lots. There were also stories of neighborhood bullies getting "taken to the cleaners" any time they gave my father trouble.

So he decided to teach me some boxing, which led to us also having boxing matches right in our driveway with any local kids who wanted to take part, a lot like he did growing up.

That tough kid up the street was more than happy to join in on the fun.

I remember feeling pretty scared facing him, but I easily beat him, bloody nose and all. He didn't really have all that aggression and anger in that match, with my father as the referee.

For some reason, I didn't feel any better about what had happened months before. So much for revenge.

Eye of the Tiger

After a few more successful fighting experiences over those early years, my confidence grew. I also learned about looking people in the eye and not being the first to look away. Basically, I learned not to back down to anyone.

With this attitude, and the fact that I would step in any time a bully was giving one of my friends a hard time, I was developing some enemies that I didn't even know about.

One of these bullies sure didn't like it, and he had all the wrong people backing him from the other side of town.

Gang Attack

At about the age of thirteen, I arrived one evening behind the schoolyard. Nothing out of the ordinary. Except this time, I saw a crowd at the far end surrounding someone on the ground.

When I got close, I could see it was my usual group of friends looking at a good friend of ours all shook up, crawling around, coughing, and throwing up.

When I asked what had happened, the group went on to tell me about how a gang of about twenty or so from the other side of town, our age and older, came through and just beat him up. They told how they surrounded him, knocked him down and punched and kicked him until they got bored.

I asked, "Did anyone help him?"

They didn't answer. This made me furious, and so disgusted with all of them. These kids were supposed to be our friends. No one had his back? No one went for help?

I learned something about people that day, and I redefined the term "friend" in my vocabulary.

Oh, and they also told me that *I was the one they were looking for*.

So he basically took the beating that was meant for me. I was even more furious.

Helping a Friend Home

It was getting dark out. As I was helping my beaten-up friend get home, we were about one block from his house when they came swarming around the corner. Clearly, they were still on their rampage.

My friend almost dropped right there and wet his pants from fear thinking he was going to get it again. He was shaking like a leaf.

They surrounded us, and as the leader and a few others approached they said to my friend, "You can go. We want him."

Which of course, was me.

A Little History

A few months back one of them had approached me at a carnival where I was told this guy wanted to fight me. I didn't even know him, but he knew me. He was apparently a friend of the local bully that I had been standing up against.

I asked him, "Why?"

He said, "I don't like your face."

I answered, "I don't like your face either, but I don't want to fight about it." And I walked away.

So, there he was again, standing next to the leader and another older kid about twice my size.

They told me I was going to fight right now, and they were nice enough to give me a choice. Either I fight the one who approached me at the carnival, or I fight the big guy.

Well, I'm no fool. Seeing no way out, I immediately turned and dumped that kid with one punch. I guess he didn't expect it. He got back up though, and after a short scuffle, I had him down on the ground and about to pummel him, when the others quickly stepped in, pulled me off and said I couldn't do that.

So now they're making up rules as we go along.

Within moments we were forced to leave by the owners of the property we were on. So they brought me to a more private setting, near my home, where we could continue.

So there we were, me and this kid I didn't even know and all his gang banger friends in a circle around us. Since there were now rules against me, it turned into sort of 'he goes, I go' and swing as hard as you can.

There was a point when a few of them took me down and started punching and kicking me. I had visions of what happened to my friend just a few short hours earlier. I said to myself, "No way!" I was able to quickly get to my feet, and I stayed focused on my main opponent.

Eventually, the sun had set, and it got dark. The big guy took out his lighter and lit it under each of our faces to check us out. He said I looked fine and asked if I was okay to continue. I said, "Sure."

When he lit up the other kid's face, it was a different picture, again like in the original Rocky movie. He asked him if he was okay to continue, and he said, "No."

Well, this infuriated the leader, who really wanted to hurt me. He was so upset that I won, that he came after me... and he was a well-known psycho who had put a few other boys in the hospital, so I didn't want to take any chances.

I broke out of the circle and just took off for home. Fortunately, I could run like a deer. No one had a chance to catch me. Just a short sprint and I was hopping over the fence at my home moments later.

Aren't some people just a joy to run into? (That's sarcasm, by the way).

There were some other situations in high school, but that was surely the most dramatic.

First Exposure to Kung Fu

I was seventeen when I first met a very influential person in my life. His name is Gerry Lopez, and years later he was the best man at my wedding. We're still very good friends to this day, and no matter how much time passes by between visits, he and I always see eye to eye.

But I'm getting ahead of myself.

Gerry was an interesting person in high school. He was quite different than most of my other friends. He was from Columbia, and when he came to this country and couldn't speak the language, he fell behind in school. He was a sixteen-year-old 9th grader.

Gerry had moved into town from Paterson, where he had been training in Shaolin Long Fist Kung Fu for about three years at the time. I was intrigued, and I asked a lot of questions.

Gerry was evasive about the whole thing. He didn't tell me much and that just added to the mystique.

I wanted him to show me some things; to teach me if he would. But he was very serious about his training and said he was not allowed to teach me anything. That was a rule.

I purchased a book called, "Shaolin Long Fist Kung Fu" by Dr. Yang Jwing-Ming that contained some of the same sequences Gerry knew. I tried to learn from the book. No luck.

Gerry told me that I was welcome to come see him in class, so I did. He called it "the Academy."

The Academy was on the edge of a pretty bad area. We entered one of the beat up old buildings and went up to the second floor where there was a small rectangular space with weapons on the wall, a few mirrors, and a bench or two to sit on. In the corner was an old big-back wicker chair that really added to the look of the place (I always loved that old chair).

I was introduced to the Shifu (Randy Elia) and then sat down to watch Gerry in his private class.

I was so impressed with the way Gerry could move. He was fluid and graceful. It was so unlike any karate I had seen in the past that was so rigid and choppy looking. These movements were more circular and blended together beautifully. Much of the practical use was not obvious by design. The Chinese were apparently very good at hiding their secrets within.

I was sold. I had a part-time job, so I worked out the tuition (had no money left for anything else), and dove in fully.

Average High School

Most everyone has had the common high school experience and know how cruel teens can be to each other, especially back in the 70's and 80's. Everyone has a label: the jocks, the heads, the nerds, the geeks, etc. Well, my experience was no different.

My friends were the jocks and boy did we think who we were. And of course, we had our post-game celebration/ parties where there was plenty of drinking going on. I even had my own stash of whiskey hidden in my car, ready for any party.

Kung Fu Training Changes Everything

It was early in 1984, my senior year, when I joined my first Kung Fu class. The year when everyone is getting the craziest, I was shifting gears.

I don't know how or why it happened, but the philosophy of the training was having a profound effect on the way I was thinking. The practice itself changed me.

There was a time when I was walking into school with a friend I'd had since the 1st grade, and at the entrance, there were a number of other kids hanging out before going inside.

He said under his breath, but where they could surely hear him, "Dirt Bags," and it was the first time in my mind it clicked. I thought, "Who are you?" and, "What makes you think you're better than they are?"

That never happened before.

That was it. I was experiencing a real shift in consciousness. I realized we all need to treat each other with respect. I realized that no one is better or worse than anyone else. I got tired of the labels and judgments and how people mock others who are not like them.

I realized we need more acceptance.

I also stopped drinking. I stopped going to the parties. There was no one telling me to. My parents didn't even know about it. I just stopped.

I went through college focused on learning, not partying, like so many around me.

I don't know how it happens, but I know from personal experience, the martial arts are a lot more than just punching, kicking, or grappling.

The Highest Level of Fighting is Not to Fight

An important message came from learning to fight. I realized the more I learned how to do it with skill the less I wanted to. I came to realize how easy it is to seriously hurt someone and with that knowledge comes responsibility. The last thing I wanted to do was hurt anybody and so learning how to avoid a fight became my mindset.

This was a big change for someone who grew up learning to use his fists to settle things.

Lessons like that and a lot more like it are what this book is all about.

Meant To Be?

Was I in the wrong place at the wrong time when that neighbor come over beat the snot out of me?

Within the first three years or so from the time I started it became clear to me that I wanted to run my own school. I was already teaching about half the classes at the Academy where I started where I was able to learn the ins and outs of running a school.

I had developed a passion for teaching what I was learning to others. It had done so much for me that I believed others would have a similar experience. I said I would have my own school within ten years.

The Phone Call

In 1993, I received a call from a person looking for someone to teach a group of CFS (chronic fatigue syndrome) patients. They had found a place - a dance school, just across the street from our current location.

There, I was able to negotiate a deal that allowed the rent to be paid based on how we grew the school. I had no money, so this was the only way it would be doable. Within a few short months, we had over 40 students, and I could drop my other jobs. I was in my tenth-year of training in Kung Fu.

When I said I would have a school in ten years, it really was an arbitrary number. But my every action was toward that goal. And the rest is history.

You never really know what may happen when you put your all into something.

Those Defining Moments

Around 1998, in addition to running my own school of martial arts, I was treating patients with Amma Therapy®, a medical massage and healing system that is based on the Oriental medical model. At this point, I did not consciously remember the beating I wrote about above. How I came to remember was while treating a woman who happened to be a known psychic (though not known to me at the time) who had done a lot of successful work for the police.

She stopped me right in the middle of a massage and gave me a reading. She told me that a very significant event happened to me at the age of 9 or 10 that changed the course of my life. She asked if I knew what it was. I didn't.

Later I remembered.

I never lost that need to have control over my self and my life. To be able to handle a situation - defend myself - if ever necessary. Now I knew where it came from.

So, what are your defining moments? What in your life experience has influenced you and landed you where you are? Is it what you really want?

If not, let's see if traditional martial arts training has something for you...

A Throwback
To Simpler Times

With same-day deliveries and YouTube videos we live in a world of instant gratification and constant distraction, the art of Kung Fu bucks the trends and provides a throwback to simpler times.

This practice provides those who apply themselves with invaluable tools and profound experiences that literally infiltrates and positively impacts everything they do.

Whatever role you take on: employee or employer, father or son, mother or daughter, brother or sister, husband or wife... this practice makes you better at it.

We have many students who've been with us five, ten, even over twenty years. Why would they still be practicing with us for so long? With all the other offerings out there why stick with one martial art, one school, and one teacher, rather than try out as much as they can? Why not go out and learn as much as they can from as many different people as they can?

It's simple: the depth that comes from quality and fully understanding the what, why, how and when versus the superficial approach of collecting techniques and ultimately becoming the "Jack of all trades and master of none."

Why do they stay so long? Because they came for one reason and stayed for something else. They experienced something they didn't expect - something profound and fulfilling - so their time with us continues - as does the positive impact on their lives.

Once you understand principles, you will find there are infinite ways to apply them in your life. It is far more than just self defense. It is also for all your many challenges in your day-to-day life.

What can be more important than the health of your body and your mind? Emotional stability? Spiritual connection?

How I Got Started & Why I'm Still At It

You've already read my story.

Like most, I came to the martial arts because I wanted to be able to fight. Or, more accurately, I wanted to be confident knowing that if I ever had to physically defend and protect myself or a loved one, I could.

However, it wasn't but a few months into training that I realized there is so much more.

And to repeat an important point, the better I became at fighting, the less interested in it I was. Why would I want to hurt someone?

Once I realized how easy it was, it became far less attractive. Besides, there were so many bigger and better things I was learning that touched every aspect of my life that the fighting became an afterthought. A means to an end.

That end was *a better life*.

I was six months into my training when I knew that it was what I wanted to dedicate my life to: Teaching and training to help make other lives better. I wanted as many people as possible to get what I was getting from this practice.

Why?

- The mental and physical training plus the integrated philosophy interwoven within the lessons completely changed my view of the world.

- I became very focused and disciplined. I virtually stopped drinking (something I did far too much of in high school) even though I was soon in college with a lot of that going on around me. The positive influence of the martial arts practice was infiltrating everything I did.
- I did far better in college than I did in high school and later, when I returned to school to study acupuncture and Chinese medicine, I found my memory and focus to be above and beyond anything I ever experienced before in education. It was... *easy!*
- I found that the ability to control a situation was rooted within. That learning to control myself, my thoughts, my actions, and reactions were the only things I really had any control over. And once I realized this I found so much more of my life seemingly to just fall into place.
- As I learned to control my mind, I became less emotional and more at peace. I found a higher level of confidence and lack of fear to try new things led to never turning down an opportunity, which opened doors I would never have seen beyond if I allowed fear and self-doubt to lead me.
- And when life hit harder from so many directions and knocked me down, as life tends to do to all of us, the resilience that resulted from my training helped me to keep getting up and continuing on.
- To this day, I'm driven not only to better myself - a never-ending pursuit - but also to help others improve their lives as well.
- To help the weak become stronger and to help the strong to develop the compassion to also help pick up those less fortunate.

- To help those filled with feelings of fear, self-doubt or unworthiness to develop a powerful presence that exudes confidence and leads to success in anything they do.
- To help people discover for themselves what they are really capable of.

Awareness:
An Essential Component
Of The Martial Artist's Practice

Martial artists train to pay attention. Awareness is an essential component of the practice. It is the number one line of self defense. But we cannot expect others to have the same level of awareness who don't train this way. In fact, in today's world, more people are more complacent about their safety and more distracted than ever.

So, it's up to you to keep yourself safe. You must be the one who is paying attention. It's not your responsibility to make others pay attention. You have no control over what others do or don't do. Getting upset or angry when others don't pay attention is a waste of your energy and doing you more harm than you realize.

Buddha said it this way:

"Holding on to anger is like grasping a hot coal with the intent of throwing it at someone else; you are the one who gets burned."

You don't even have to be affected by what others do or don't do. You only have to be aware of when you need to respond. If a car is coming at you, get out of the way. It's as simple as that. No need to get emotional about it.

IT'S A POWERFUL LIFE

As a teacher, I'm frequently reminding students of the importance of awareness and that this practice is 24/7. A martial artist is always practicing. There is no down time.

If someone doesn't show you respect do you get upset? Do you become angry? Do you see them as a bad person?

Certainly, you're human, and you may frequently respond emotionally, but you don't have to hold on to that emotion.

A car is coming toward you. You jump out of the way. Your adrenaline is flowing, and you feel fear coursing through your veins. You may even come to tears.

Are you safe now? If so, move on. Drop it. Let it go and forget about it. That's how it works in the natural world, the world of Dao.

However, because we're so smart, we tend to make it more than it is. We can tell that story and relive that terrible experience for years to come.

And that, once you understand it, is a choice.

I will expand on this throughout the book. For some specific chapters go to Part Four: "A Lifetime of Return on Investment" and the discussion of personal safety in the Addendum.

PART ONE

What's Holding You Back?

I've been teaching martial arts for over thirty years. I've taught all kinds of people from the age of eight to over eighty, and my wife teaches them as young as three.

I've seen thousands of students come and go over the years. Some stick it out and have been with us over ten or even twenty years. Some stop as life gets in the way but then return because they love the practice.

What I've found is a common theme of why they come:

- They like to be active and in shape, but they're bored and tired of the usual one-dimensional exercises they get at the gym.
- They struggle with time. In today's world, we're all so busy with so many responsibilities that finding time for ourselves is becoming more and more difficult.
- They're stressed, looking for an outlet. They want to learn how to relax. They want to feel calmer and more settled.
- They'd like to feel more confident. They believe that this lack of confidence, feelings of fear and self-doubt, is holding them back in their careers, relationships, and life in general.
- They would like to be more focused and disciplined. They tend to procrastinate and would like to change that about themselves so they can better pursue their dreams.
- They also tend to have an attraction to the martial arts, always wanted to pursue it, but thought it may be too hard or they might get hurt.

Does any of this describe you? If so, keep reading...

CHAPTER I

---◆━━━━◆---

You're Bored With the Gym and Your One-Dimensional Exercise

If you're bored with your exercise routine, you're not likely to keep it up. Consider, running on a treadmill vs. training your whole body and mind. Most people believe that anything that gets their heart rate up is exercise and that exercise is all about the heart. But these long bouts of cardio have been found to actually be a negative for some people! Did you know that many marathon runners have damaged their heart?

The ancient Chinese philosophical approach to life is to strive to be as close to natural laws as possible. One concept that came out of this is that we only have so many heartbeats. Preserving those heartbeats helps to promote a longer, healthier life. We weren't built to run long distances like marathons or engage in regular endurance training. The heart cannot handle the volume of blood that must move through it for that kind of demand. In fact, endurance training or long bouts of cardio have been shown to have the same effect as a heart attack!

According to Colin E. Champ, M.D., in his book, "Misguided Medicine": "Many physicians are now regularly seeing 50-year-old male joggers with evidence of heart damage and an irregular heartbeat."

Citing a study by La Gerche A., Burns AT, and Mooney DJ, entitled, "Exercise-induced right ventricular dysfunction and structural remodeling in endurance athletes," Dr. Champ's book discusses how long bouts of cardio have been shown to increase inflammation of the heart and decrease blood flow to the heart itself, resulting in damage. The heart must adapt to this demand and become bigger and thicker which results in a dysfunctional pump for your whole cardiovascular system. This change in the heart also has a negative effect on breathing as it puts pressure on the lungs.

In my experience feeling thousands of pulses over the years, from a Chinese perspective, I have found just as many poor readings of the heart in athletes as in non-athletes. I have not found that the athletes who are running numerous miles per week, or training for and competing in "Ironman"-type competitions, show any indication of benefit to their heart. In fact, I find the opposite is true, and research consistent with this continues at the largest Chinese medical clinic in the country led by one Robert Doane, EAMP, L.Ac., Dipl.C.H., in Poulsbo, Washington.

Aging Faster Too?

In her article, "Does Cardio Exercise Make A Person Age?" Janine Grant writes, "Moderate cardio might actually slow aging by conditioning your body to adapt to stress. By contrast, signs of aging such as loss of lean body mass, increased belly fat, oxidative stress, inflammation and heart damage could be a potential consequence of excessive cardio."

The jury is still out about cardio and aging and what is "excessive" differs from person to person. Diet, sleep, stress and other factors must be considered as well.

However, if I can get the same or even better health and fitness benefit in a much shorter amount of time why not take advantage?

You could be doing various fun, practical martial arts skills and drills. Built into the workout could be strength and mobility exercises that take into account your whole body and mind. Or, you can keep doing those long, boring, steady-state cardio workouts, (like running on a treadmill for an hour or more).

Ultimately, all this time and effort *for* your health may actually be making you *less* healthy and age faster. Sort of defeats the purpose of exercise, don't you think?

Exercising the Natural Way

I've had some amazing experiences in the wilderness with courses given by Tom Brown, Jr. at his Tracker School, and his student, Jon Young, when he would visit the Vermont Wilderness School. Plus my own "dirt time" applying what they taught about survival, tracking and essentially living as native peoples did all over the world for millions of years: as "hunter-gatherers." Just like those who hunted and gathered their food, we did plenty of walking, digging, squatting, crawling, crouching under brush, climbing, and carrying heavy things in those courses.

A burst of speed to catch what was hunted or to escape a predator were all common daily activities for our ancestors. (According to accounts of people such as anthropologist Dr. Kim Hill, who spent a lot of time with the Ache people of Eastern Paraguay.)

In fact, and as I often joke in classes when discussing this topic, native people have no toilets – so everyone was excellent at squatting!

Squatting is a natural human movement, one that has been lost due simply to a lack of use. But you can get it back.

Much of how we've used our bodies over millions of years is used in some way in traditional Chinese martial arts, or Kung Fu, training, as well as other martial arts from the Far East, where mimicking animals was a factor in its development. These arts were developed over thousands of years not only for the battlefield but also to promote health, longevity, strength and mobility.

These arts are based on what's most natural and even necessary for us to perform regularly for optimal health and wellbeing.

The human body has many different muscles, tendons, ligaments, joints, and other body structures and systems such as your organs, circulatory system, nervous system, lymphatic system, digestive system.

Warm up exercises should be focused on whole body mobility, hitting each joint from multiple angles so you can maintain the range of motion you're supposed to have, not simply to break a sweat and raise the heart rate (which is automatic with proper mobility work). It should also mimic what you plan to do more intensely during training.

Qigong (pronounced "chee gung") training, which is like a slow, moving meditation and a traditional component of Chinese martial arts, promotes increased circulation of healing "Qi and blood" throughout the body.

Qi (pronounced, "chee") in this context is the oxygen we get from the air and the nutrients we get from food. Optimal health is when this Qi and blood circulates unencumbered to reach every cell in the body. Any place that is not reached leads to dysfunction or disease of that area of the body.

Highly sophisticated Qigong training is simple to learn and fully designed with these principles in mind.

Martial Arts Skills Training is Exercise.

You don't need to practice your skills and then find more time for cardio. In fact, as you'll soon see, shorter more intense bursts of exercise are actually healthier and more effective.

Only the right exercise (for you) done with the proper frequency, duration, and intensity (also specific to you) will have the greatest impact on your health, strength, and mobility. Get it wrong or be misled, and you'll either not make progress, or you're an injury waiting to happen.

Repetitive movements are known to cause injury. This is even more true when you don't move well.

You're exercising so you can be healthier, and now you're in pain!

For example, as much as they love it, it is very common for runners to experience a lot of leg, knee and back pain as they age. Is it the wrong amount? Wrong technique? Wrong footwear? The repetitive pounding with each step? What?

With proper training that includes proper body mechanics, you can learn to move with ease, age with grace, and keep in phenomenal shape.

You can feel young forever.

CHAPTER 2

You Don't Have Much Time

Learn how to save time by getting more out of less.

If you use a multi-faceted approach to health and fitness, you'll find more ways to benefit in less time. That's efficiency.

Meditation is the foundation of all true martial arts and I recommend that students meditate every day. You want to be a martial artist? You must meditate every day. Period.

Your first reaction to that may be, "I don't have time to meditate!"

I understand.

However, without going into the many benefits of regular meditation that are now widely known (and easily "Googled"), once you understand *how to meditate* you'll soon learn that *everything we do here is meditation.*

And it can be taken into every moment of your life. I'll elaborate a little more in a moment.

Shorter "Workouts" While Getting More Out of Them.

As already explained above, the long bouts with jogging, running on treadmills, or mimicking ironman (or woman) workouts are a thing of the flawed recent past. Studies are showing that not only did our native ancestors never engage in endurance exercise, shorter more intense exercise (like a sprint from danger) actually has the greatest overall effect.

Do you really need those 60-90 minute grueling cardio/endurance sessions 3-4 times per week, weight training another 60-90 minutes 3 times per week on your "off days" from cardio, plus yoga, meditation and Pilates to round things out, **leaving you too exhausted to really give your all the rest of the day** (and confirming what you now know *may not be so good for you after all!*)?

Then There's Travel Time...

Do you need to go to multiple locations or class times (doing your best to fit the gym schedule into yours), battle traffic, struggle to find parking and a locker to put your stuff so you can get in your cardio, Pilates, yoga, meditation, and strength training? You've heard they're all good so you want it all, right?

Have you done the math here for how much time is really involved?

Training Smart

A lot can be accomplished all in one place when training in traditional martial arts. How about training smart an hour 2-3 times per week? Your time at the training hall, *dojang**, or *dojo** might include:

- A short sitting meditation to get you in the moment, focused and mentally prepared to learn

37

- A full body mobility session (that all counts toward your "workout" time) that over time will completely change your body from stiff to supple in ten minutes
- Fun traditional martial arts skills training that not only gets you in great shape but develops more focus and coordination
- Specially designed and integrated bodyweight training that builds strength, mobility, and secretly teaches you how to move far more efficiently and effectively (while saving your lower back!)
- Partner training (where you work *with* each other rather than *against!*) to hammer home the lesson, develop more focus, timing, distance and reaction skills while you learn practical self defense *that could save your life one day!*
- Ending with traditional "martial qigong" to further enhance your developing skills while you cool down and coordinate your movements with your breathing and concentration
- And all of it can be a meditation. An essential part of the training is to focus only on what you're doing in the moment and be fully engaged. The greatest effects on your body and your life will be when your mind and body are working together. (No running on a treadmill while watching TV!)

Which gets in all you need to stay healthy, strong, mobile, and focused while energizing instead of exhausting you.

For those who really want to get good at this, simply do a little on your own 1-2 days per week *anytime or anywhere you please!*

It's a School!

You get a real education for your body and your mind with traditional martial arts training with the added benefit that if it's ever a problem for you to get to class, although you may prefer to train with a group, *you don't always have to*. Again, you'll be able to train anytime, anywhere.

And you'll learn how this practice permeates all areas of your life and everything you do. These are lessons you won't forget.

*See Chapter 12: Find Your Special *Place* for an explanation of these terms.

CHAPTER 3

—◆——◆——

Stress and Anxiety:
It's Hard To Relax

Exercise is known to reduce stress, help you relax more easily and sleep better too.

Meditation is known to raise the threshold for stress so you can handle stress more easily.

Put five people in the same bad situation, and you'll get five different responses: some break down, others thrive and are able to pick others up. You can be the one who thrives.

Breathing: The Bridge Between the Body and Mind

- The breath can relax your body
- The breath can calm your mind.

Once you understand how it works think all the challenges and stressful moments in your life. How would it feel to be able to simply turn to a breathing technique you've learned in class and get your body and mind on your side when you need them most?

Change How You See Things

Traditional martial arts are rooted in meditation and breath control techniques. A calm mind is a capable mind. It is able to help you be more productive and creative. It also helps you to change how you see things. And that's the real secret to changing your life.

Through the practice of traditional Kung Fu, and the eastern philosophy that it has always been integrated with, you'll learn to see things differently. You'll realize that the only thing you can control is yourself. You cannot control the world around you or make others change. Simply realizing this and learning to recognize and accept things as they are can greatly reduce stress and bring profound peace in your life.

It simply makes life more enjoyable.

Facing Adversity

One thing that good martial arts training includes that few other things do is facing adversity. You could say that sports can have this effect, but that's based on winning and losing: someone has to feel like they're better than someone else (be it one-on-one or with a team) and when they discover otherwise this is considered adversity.

The only adversity that counts in our lives is what's going on within. Your only real competition in life *is yourself*.

The basic premise of Kung Fu is about overcoming one's self-imposed limiting beliefs *a little at a time*.

We get stressed and anxious when things don't go the way we want them to or happen when we want them to. That's what holds us back in life. We change course and many times end up never getting anywhere we really want to be.

Facing adversity like this strengthens both the body and the mind in a way that makes lives better.

A strong body and mind is like having a bigger cup: you can take on a lot more before it becomes too much.

CHAPTER 4

Fear and Self-Doubt / Lack of Confidence

How many things have you not pursued in your life because of fear? How is fear holding you back in your career? Could you be moving up faster? Be making more money? Getting better results? Enjoying better relationships?

When you're run by fear and self-doubt, it has a negative impact on your life: your job or career, the money you make, the relationships you have, etc.

With poor focus, low energy, and constant anxiety, how can you expect to be your best at work or at play? Or to be a good partner to someone? How can you be able to listen and understand their wants or fears? You can't. And that puts a strain on any relationship.

Was it fear of failure? Fear of what others might think? Fear of getting hurt? How much have you missed out on because of it? Being run by fear makes your world very small and limited. What might you be missing out on because of fear?

We're afraid of things we aren't familiar with. Confidence can only come from personal experience. How can you possibly be the confident person you want to be if you avoid new things and don't expand on your experiences? You can't.

You CAN overcome your fears and have the confidence to pursue your dreams. You just have to step up and be willing to do the work.

Self-Limiting Beliefs

When your world gets smaller due to fear or lack of confidence, it can really suck the life out you! When you're so caught up in thinking you are somehow better or worse than others, does that lead to healthy relationships?

Are you easily insulted?

Developing toughness and thicker skin will allow you to go all out for the things you want in life and not be so concerned with results. It may seem contradictory, but it is not. What holds you back is thinking or worrying about failing, falling, or even making a fool of yourself.

These are all internal problems that hold you back. It's not the world... it's you.

But that's good news! Because *you* are all you can control. Your thoughts, your words, your actions, and reactions are all you can really do anything about.

When you get passed these imagined negative outcomes, or essentially aren't affected by them even if they do occur, then you can attack your life with all you've got. THAT is guaranteed to get better results than not even trying because of what *might* happen or what you believe others may think.

When you start doing what it takes to overcome these self-imposed limitations and begin to realize what you're capable of you won't care what others think or say. You'll do what you choose to do with your time and your life.

Crippling People By Doing Too Much For Them.

If we don't allow our children or our loved ones to do for themselves - to fail and fall down by their own efforts or lack thereof - they will never develop the necessary resilience to overcome adversity and challenges. They will not learn what they are capable of or believe in themselves. If they don't earn their keep so to speak, they will not be able to. There will be no self-esteem.

And when life gets hard they will get frustrated and depressed. Pills are not the answer. Stepping up and actually *doing something* for themselves is.

There's a saying, "Fall down seven times, stand up eight." That's the attitude and approach of those who've trained themselves in traditional martial arts.

Your only competition is yourself.

CHAPTER 5

Lack of Focus and Discipline

Another saying: "Do what you have to do then you can do what you want to do."

How you use your time is a habit: Discipline or lack of discipline - both are habits.

A focused mind spends less energy. It's less distracted and calmer.

You CAN Be More Focused.

Do you complain that you don't have enough time? When you're unfocused, it only gets worse as you are all over the place running like a mouse on a wheel making so much effort and getting nowhere at all. You feel like you don't get anything done. Or you feel like you get a lot done but there's always more!

With a focus in one direction at a time, you'll be amazed at your progress and how your life changes.

You CAN Be More Disciplined.

You know what you should do, but you don't do it. Lacking the discipline to do what needs to be done so you can get where you want to go in life will result in life continuing to pass you by.

Time stops for no one. Six weeks, six months, or six years will go by whether you pursue your dreams or not.

You can feel like that mouse on a wheel, working hard, struggling, and getting nowhere as you juggle too many things. Or, you can get focused on one road and make real progress in your life.

Focus on the right thing - the one thing that helps to improve everything else, and your time and energy will be well spent. You'll be amazed at how much your life changes for the better.

When we focus on something, it is like turning up the volume. Whatever we focus on is amplified.

Have a problem? Focus on it, and you will experience an emotional downword spiral.

Focus on the solution - *what can you do about this problem?* And watch the possibilities come to you. There may be many viable options you wouldn't have considered if you continued to be caught up in the "Oh my God!...," "I can't believe...," "Why me?..." and other unhelpful thoughts that only serve to keep you stuck and suffering.

Focus and discipline take practice. Each is like a weak muscle, unable to complete the task at hand until strengthened through consistent use.

Real martial artists have trained their minds and their bodies. They are focused. They are disciplined.

You can be too.

Try This:

A Simple Exercise
For Better Concentration

Before you can meditate, you must be able to concentrate. "The Concentration Exercise," as it was referred to by my Shifu, Grandmaster Park, is like a prerequisite to meditation.

To start, visualize a number in your mind. 50 is a good place to start, but some may want to start with 20. The goal is to count backward in your mind, seeing each number as clearly as you can, and holding it in your mind's eye for about 3-5 seconds, before going on to the next number. Just sort of see the shape as you imagine each number. Take notice how often you lose track, or you may even start again when you do to challenge yourself. See how many attempts it takes to get to zero without losing track.

When you reach zero, you are finished with the exercise and may just continue to sit quietly until it becomes uncomfortable. How long? That depends on you. If it is causing stress, then it is too long.

Shifu Park said that when he learned from his Shifu, he had to be able to go from 500 to zero without losing track or having the mind wander. Only then would he be taught how to meditate!

Many people sit and believe they are meditating, but their minds are all over the place without them realizing it. This exercise is a way to gauge progress quite well. However, don't get caught up in how you're doing. Simply, practice. Like lifting weights to get stronger, you must progress gradually and enjoy the process.

It is interesting to note how the Concentration Exercise naturally leads one to focus on the third eye point. As you visualize, it is as if you are creating a mental screen where you see the numbers.

In the Bhagavad Gita, it says, "...through devotion and the power of meditation, with your mind completely stilled and your concentration fixed in the center of spiritual awareness between the eyebrows, you will realize the Supreme."

In mind research conducted by Jose Silva, creator of the Silva Method, he found that closing the eyes and looking about 20 degrees upward would trigger the brain into what is known as Alpha (a much calmer, focused state).

For some, numbers may be stressful. If numbers are something you work with all day, like a bookkeeper or accountant, then it may not be the way to go for you. Other visualizations that we use are designed to create a good feeling inside and known as "Happiness Meditations."

There are specific instructions we use for these, but simply focusing on something natural and alive that results in a happy feeling will suffice here.

Don't "See" It?

Occasionally, a student will ask what to do if they can't "see" anything in their mind's eye. They may say, "I can't visualize."

First, saying that you "can't" about anything, puts up a road block that will make it impossible.

Second, if I ask you to describe your dog, cat, car, etc. could you do it? If you say your car is green, and it is outside where you can't physically see it, then how do you know it's green? Did you memorize the letters, "g-r-e-e-n?" Of course not. You saw it in your mind. We all think with images.

Some are certainly more visual than others, and will find it easier, but everyone can visualize - it's just a matter of concentration. Your ability to focus - control your mind - is essentially the foundation of the whole practice of martial arts. It is worth the time to work on it, just as we do with any skill.

PART TWO

How You Can Easily Have More
Energy, Better Health, Less Stress,
and Live a More Powerful Life

If you want to learn how to play music, you must first learn each note. You then learn how to combine these notes and play beautiful sounds that others have created.

Eventually, the best create their own.

If you want to learn how to read, you must start with the alphabet. The letters are strung together to make words, then sentences, paragraphs, and books.

The best created great literary works for you to read.

Once you know the basic rules and enough words, you could even create your own.

Most martial arts are a collection of techniques that once the student remembers, they feel like they know something. They are then tested and progress in rank.

Maybe they compete and earn a collection of trophies to show off.

In a few years, they may even earn a black belt and feel like they have accomplished something.

Are the martial arts all about tournaments, trophies, and black belts?

For some, that may be true.

However, what is offered in this book goes above and beyond that superficial level and into a never-ending practice that teaches us how to:

- live fully, in the moment
- maintain excellent health
- feel energetic, happy, and satisfied
- age gracefully
- enjoy a calm and peaceful state of mind
- be confident and true to yourself

It's a practice that makes you stronger mentally, emotionally and physically, as well as more connected spiritually, so you are better equipped to handle whatever life throws your way.

Here are the principles of an ancient Chinese martial art, based on natural laws, to know and live by...

CHAPTER 6

If You Give A Man A Fish...

L et me tell you the story of two very different fathers.
The first one loved his family so much that he would get up very early in the morning, hours before the sunrise when it was still very dark, even in the cold of winter, so that he could be out in the water to catch fish. It is in these early morning hours that the fish are hungry and looking for food.

Also, the fish markets opened very early, so he would have to catch and then carry his fish to the market before the first customers arrived. This is how he made his living and fed his family. It was a difficult start to his day, but he did it every morning before his family even woke up because he loved them so much.

The young son of the first father had a good friend whose father was also a fisherman.

The second father was very different. He would awaken his young son and make him come along for these same difficult early morning outings, even in the cold of winter. He would make his young son catch the fish, carry it to the market, and

IF YOU GIVE A MAN A FISH...

even clean it and prepare it for the family. The young boy really hated these early morning chores and wished his father was more like his friend's father.

One day the military came through and recruited all able-bodied men for the war. Both fathers had to go, and unfortunately, both died in the war.

Which family was now better off?

The second father loved his family so much that he made sure they were able to take care of themselves when he was no longer there to do it for them.

A bird must eventually leave the nest and fly on its own. A child must one day make their own way in this world as an adult. A student must eventually be able to figure things out for him or herself and move on independent of the teacher.

Sometimes the bird is kicked out of the nest and forced to fly. Sometimes the parent must kick their adult child out of the house, forcing them to make their own way.

Is the bird, the child, and the student ready? Have they been properly prepared?

The bird will fly just as the baby will walk by the natural process and sheer determination.

The student, however, just as the son in the fisherman story above, must be taught in a way that leads to independence for when the teacher, like the father, is no longer there.

And so there is the saying, "Give a man a fish, you feed him for a day; teach a man to fish, and you feed him for a lifetime."

CHAPTER 7

—◆—————◆—

Move With Meaning

I've always been most interested in getting the best results for both my students and myself.

I have a long-standing interest in keeping up with the world of exercise and fitness. I have a degree in exercise physiology as well as certifications that include the Russian Kettlebell (StrongFirst Level 2) and the CSCS (Certified Strength and Conditioning Specialist from the NSCA).

I find that this background, along with a healthy obsession with proper movement mechanics (due to the various physical challenges I've experienced - and was able to correct - over the years) makes me better equipped to be able to transfer the ancient knowledge of the body and mind of traditional Kung Fu to modern day students of the martial arts in a way that results in the most effective and efficient approach to training possible.

Ultimately what differentiates a martial arts training program from your average gym rat and the "workout of the day" scenario is that the movements are skill-based versus whatever it takes to get you moving, sweating and working your butt off to look good on the beach or in the bedroom.

Skill-based training has a purpose beyond just getting you in shape or making you look good (though still results in those things). Proper training in the various arts of Kung Fu automatically gets you in great shape, while increasing strength and mobility.

This training also enhances balance as well as mental focus and discipline. And not to be forgotten: the ability to not only physically defend yourself but also the tools necessary to avoid the physical attack or confrontation altogether.

The real goal in self defense is to avoid the situation. If that isn't possible or it's too late, the next goal is to get out of the situation as quickly and safely as possible. That's very different than beating your adversary to a pulp.

Hopefully, no one gets hurt.

CHAPTER 8

Make This Shift In Your Approach and Your Life Will Never Be the Same

There are so many ways to practice martial arts. There's punching, kicking, ground fighting, stick fighting, knife fighting, etc.

There are those who focus on competition where tournaments and trophies are what it's all about.

Whether it's kickboxing, MMA, pay-per-view events or underground, the overall focus is somehow on winning and being better than others.

Besides being all about the ego, this approach is primarily *technique based*: knowing more techniques is equated with high levels, or having won more tournaments with the trophies to show for it is the sign of success.

Are the martial arts all about the ego boost? Is it just about fighting, winning (or losing), and competition? It is, if we're only discussing the *sports* side of the martial arts world.

However, traditional martial arts tend to follow the *Dao De Jing*, as it states in Chapter 66:

"The wise person does not compete, therefore, no one can compete with him (or her)."

The traditional martial artist is always striving to become "a wise person." His concerns are not about what others are doing or not doing. Her only focus is on improving herself.

This is the angle I present. It is one that I do believe is why traditional martial arts have endured over hundreds and even thousands of years and been passed down from generation to generation.

A Basic Blueprint

Of course, we need a basic blueprint to start from. We need proven techniques and drills that are known to work if self defense is the main concern.

However, we also need proven techniques to cover other important skills in life, such as self-discipline, self-control, calmness, compassion, empathy, gratitude and respect, just to name a few. Not having this skill set may be why there is so much fighting in the first place.

Why shouldn't one's martial arts training include these other aspects that may very well be far more important?

The Military Influence...

Using military training as a related example, recruits must successfully complete their bootcamp. This is known to be a very difficult challenge, both mentally and physically, also designed to weed out those who do not belong and are not fit to be a soldier.

Physically, their bodies must be built up to handle the tasks expected of a soldier. Their muscles, tendons, and ligaments must be conditioned right along with their cardiovascular endurance.

Let's not forget at some point they are going to be handed a gun. Actually, an assault rifle. We know all too well the death and devastation these weapons can lead to in the wrong hands.

Are they mentally and emotionally ready to respond appropriately with that deadly weapon in hand? Do they respect what the weapon is capable of? Do they highly value and have a healthy respect for human life? Any life?

Will they turn to it only if absolutely necessary or use it inappropriately with a knee-jerk emotional reaction at the drop of a hat?

These are questions that must seriously be considered and appropriately addressed.

For one thing, are they highly trained in diffusion? Can they maintain their heads and stop a violent threat without turning to violence themselves and making things worse?

There must be so much more to their training. Military personnel are taught to maintain their gear, their living quarters, and themselves to the highest standards.

They are known to be highly disciplined. When in a group, they must be fully aware of each other. When in lines, those lines better well be perfectly straight.

You know this. I'm sure you've seen it for yourself, if not in person, then on TV or in movies.

Every bit of it serves a purpose.

This is the way of the martial artist as well. To hold themselves to the highest standards. To take their responsibilities seriously and perform to the absolute best of their ability.

Martial arts training is rooted in ancient military discipline. That's why we say Kung Fu is not a sport, *it's a discipline.*

The discipline, focus, and confidence, as well as their general physical preparedness, are all a part of what it means to be a martial artist.

The martial artist maintains their body and their mind so they are better equipped to handle whatever life throws at them, from the loss of a job or loved one to the extreme active shooter situations we hear far too much about in today's world.

The martial artist is steady; mentally and emotionally. They are prepared mentally, emotionally, and physically.

They have to be.

CHAPTER 9

Ancient Theories in Modern
Days

The martial art style I've practiced for the last thirty years plus is called, *Ba Gua Zhang*, (literally, "Eight Trigrams Palm"). It is a Chinese martial art that records have attributed to one Dong Hai Chuan as the first to make it public around the mid to late 1800's. It may be much older, though nobody knows for sure.

One thing we know to be true is that the style was named for philosophical concepts that are based on natural laws. For thousands of years, these theories have been developed by sages who lived in and observed the natural world.

They called it, *Dao* (道, or *Tao*, depending on which Romanization of Chinese characters you prefer).

A literal translation of the word is, "the Way," like a road or path. This path is considered one that is in line with the laws of nature.

Anything that is inconsistent with or against nature is considered off the path, not the Way, or simply not in accordance with the Dao. Being out of line with the Dao is believed to result in everything from difficulty to disease and death.

Yin and Yang, Wuxing (Five Elements or Phases), and Ba Gua (Eight Trigrams)

My teacher for 25 years, Grandmaster Bok-Nam Park, called these the "Trinity of Natural Principles." The word trinity is used because all three work as one. Each aspect is required. If one is missing the whole system breaks down and there would be no life.

For example, Yin and Yang can be night and day, respectively. The Wuxing would then be morning (Wood), midday (Fire), afternoon (Earth), evening (Metal), and night (Water), which cycles through and repeats. The Ba Gua represents the many varied possibilities within the continuous changing from Yin to Yang to Yin... (night to day to night...) and so on.

Temperature changes would be a good example. Although there are some consistencies (morning and evening tend to be cooler than midday), there are no hard rules. The Farmer's Almanac was able to be quite accurate based on natural cycles. However, there are endless fluctuations. Weathermen (or women), even with all their modern meteorological education and equipment, still often get it wrong!

Because it is always changing.

Sometimes it gets warmer toward the evening. Sometimes it rains, Sometimes it snows. Sometimes it's windy.

Although there are repeating cycles, everything is constantly changing. This is the Principle of Change. It is the actual meaning of the Ba Gua.

The Yi Jing (I Ching)

The book where this concept originated was written over 5000 years ago and is known as the *Yi Jing*, or "Classic of Changes." This is where the Ba Gua comes from. It may be the oldest surviving book in the world.

The Yi Jing has been used for thousands of years for everything from fortune telling to medicine to general guidance on how to live in balance with all things, from the natural world to the people in our lives.

How does this relate to the practice of martial arts?

According to Daoist concepts, we are a microcosm of the macrocosm. In other words, our bodies must follow the same rules as everything else in nature.

For example, if I want to water my lawn I can use a sprinkler. If I turn on the water and find there is no water pressure at the sprinkler, even though the water may be turned on all the way, clearly something is wrong. Most likely somewhere along the hose is a bend or kink and it blocks the flow of the water from fully reaching the sprinkler. The flow there is weak, even though the source is strong.

This is no different than having what people refer to as a "pinched nerve" making numbness or pain. Although the nerve may not actually be physically pinched, the flow (or signal) is blocked or impeded, usually from muscle tension but sometimes from something structural.

This can also happen to any other part of the body. If there is poor circulation to any part of the body, that part won't be able to function properly. The cells won't be able to "eat" or "breathe" or eliminate waste. The area will break down or degenerate and most likely become painful or diseased. It could be an organ like your heart or liver, or it can be your shoulder, lower back, hip, or knee.

Similarly, think of when a river has been dammed and rerouted to bring water where we want it. Anything downstream that was once doing very well will now dry up and likely die.

The opposite where there is an abrupt change in elevation or when a larger, wider river meets a narrower channel. These changes result in a faster more powerful water flow. Also, changes in shapes of the river bed by erosion at varying rates (depending on the hardness of rocks) affect the water flow causing rapids.

In the river, the greater the change (gradient, width, erosion), the more pronounced the effect. It is the more abrupt change from the norm that brings the power. It is the contrast of Yin and Yang.

Our bodies work the same way. It is one thing to be tense (and block the flow of blood) or to be relaxed (and allow the blood to flow freely). It is when we move in a way that creates increased tension followed by deeper and more complete relaxation that the blood flow becomes much stronger.

Think of the water of a great river as it meets a dam. There are great forces that the dam must hold back. If we release the dam, or it breaks somehow, the water will flow with great power for a while. You wouldn't want to be standing in front of it at that moment!

Soon, however, the flow of the river would calm down and return to normal.

We make a dam within our bodies with tension and when this tension is released the blood flow increases. It will flow stronger than it does normally where there is no tension. Then, just like the river, it will quickly return to normal.

It is the *contrast*, the change from Yang (tension) to Yin (relaxation) that results in a strong sensation that can easily be felt by the practitioner.

All we have to do now to direct more flow of Qi (oxygen and nutrients) and blood to where it is needed (such as a problem area) is understand what part of the body, or which joints, need to move.

For overall health and enhanced cardiovascular function, this tells us that all we have to do is regularly and even systematically move as many parts of the body through their full range of motion as we can.

The concept of Ba Gua is applied here to the body as we create change through the use of the joints. In order to move, we must use a joint. The muscles, tendons, ligaments, and neurological connections work automatically. You only need to decide to move, the brain does the rest by sending the message. Generally, this is a pretty simple procedure, and the art of Ba Gua Zhang teaches a systematic way to make the most out of your efforts.

In the next section, we're going touch on this.

CHAPTER 10

Recharging Your Battery

Your body is a lot like that mobile device you carry around. The more you use it, the faster the battery runs out and needs to be recharged. You wake up in the morning with a full charge (hopefully!) just like your phone that was plugged in overnight.

Our mobile devices (smartphones, etc.) are about 30 times more powerful than the supercomputers of just twenty years ago. Do you realize what your brain is capable of? It is estimated that the human brain *is still about 30 times more powerful than today's most powerful supercomputers!* This is according to the AI Impacts project, created by two PhD students, Paul Christiano and Katja Grace, from the University of California, Berkeley, and Carnegie Mellon University, respectively.

Picture this: one hundred billion cells, each with up to ten thousand individual connections to other cells! According to the article in Scientific American, "What is the Memory Capacity of the Human Brain?" by Paul Reber, it has the storage capacity of three million hours of TV shows. Reber estimates the "brain's memory storage capacity to be something closer to around 2.5 petabytes." One petabyte equals one million gigabytes! He says, "You would have to leave the TV running continuously for more than 300 years to use up all that storage."

That's a lot.

Just Like A Car…

A car has two fuel sources. If the battery is dead, the starter cannot make a spark to ignite the gas.

The battery is Yin (internal). The gas is Yang (external). (I don't mean to confuse things here, but I do want to mention that Yin and Yang are relative, not absolute. I could easily say it's the other way around depending on perspective: the initiating spark is Yang and the substance that is burned (fuel) like food would then be Yin. But let's keep it simple for now!)

As you know, we do not see the air we breathe. We only know that we must inhale this invisible force. At least that's the way it appeared to the ancients. Before modern discoveries of what is actually in the air, the Chinese saw it as *Qi*.

We know now that oxygen is the essential element that sustains life and thin air would be considered to have "less Qi." By any name, it is obvious when we find that we cannot breathe such as when miners get trapped. The oxygen only lasts so long in stagnant air. We cannot see it, but we can definitely feel it.

We can survive about three weeks without food and about one week without water (depending on conditions).

However, more than five minutes without air and that's about all she wrote.

Clearly, the most essential element is oxygen.

The brain weighs only about two-and-a-half to three pounds. That's about 2% of the average sized person. Yet, 15-20% of the blood pumped by the heart goes to this one organ. Four arteries feed the head while only two arteries feed both of the much larger legs (one each).

The brain uses about 20-30% of the total calories you take in and 25% of your total oxygen intake. Overall, the brain uses about ten times more energy than the rest of the body.

The information processing units of the brain are neurons. As these neurons fire, they need to be constantly recharged. The more they fire, the more energy is consumed and subsequently needed to be replenished.

Now think about your life. What demands are you placing on your brain with your day-to-day activities and responsibilities? How much is necessary and how much is wasted?

The more thoughts, worries, fears, guilt, distractions, and other mental gymnastics you have to perform throughout your day, the less energy you have for anything else.

What this means is that you have less energy available to perform the trillions of metabolic processes that must continuously occur within your body to keep you healthy and strong.

And then there's what you are actually consciously doing in the moment at hand... such as driving, which becomes a very dangerous endeavor if you're not fully paying attention (over 40,000 lives lost every year on U.S. roads).

Continuous Recharging...
We are constantly replenishing the oxygen in our system since breathing is continuous. The thing is we are simply spending too much. It is one thing to recharge, however, what we really need is to "unplug" ourselves. In other words, spend less.

There are two ways to build up your bank account: one is to work and put some away regularly; the other is to spend less (and therefore save more). If you do both, increase your income and spend less, your bank account will grow much faster (and you'll feel a lot less stress about all those bills!).

Proper nourishment with quality foods, good breathing habits, and meditation accomplishes exactly that. It all adds up to a body that is vibrant and full of energy for living.

Then you can have more energy for digestion, healing, playing and anything else your life requires of you. If you can "do what you're doing" and not have so much extra energy wasted, leaking out with all the additional thoughts, worries, and other distractions, you will not only feel better and have more energy, but you'll also perform better at whatever task you have at hand.

You'll feel more energetic, less stressed, and enjoy life more.

CHAPTER 11

Use It or Lose It

Have you ever been out in nature and came upon a murky pond? It looks dark and dirty, and you really don't want to go swimming in there. Still water harbors disease. You'll see a lot more growth of bacteria and algae. These are the same things that are treated with chemicals such as chlorine to kill off all this growth and make swimming pool water look clear.

On the other hand, a river flowing powerfully will wash itself out, sending everything downstream. Even though we have polluted the waters over most of the planet, it is the moving waters that are cleanest, clearest, and support the most life. Just compare the difference of moving water (like a river) with still water (like a pond) for yourself.

Your body is the same. Your blood must circulate strongly throughout and reach every cell. Every cell must breathe, every cell must eat, and every cell must eliminate waste.

If any of this is hindered, illness, injury, and disease are certain.

And when you show up at your doctor's office in your mid to late thirties complaining of any or all these new aches, pains, stiffness, anxiety, sleeping difficulties, fatigue, and headaches, that you "never had before," you're sure to get the canned answer:

"Well, you *are* getting older..."

Think again of the powerful flow of a river. After a storm, it can increase significantly which would, in turn, wash away just about anything that is "sticking" during normal flow rates. Our circulatory system works like this as well, and modern research continues to improve our understanding of this: short, intense bursts of exercise have a far greater positive impact on health than the long "steady-state" exercise (like 60-90 minutes on a treadmill) still recommended by many doctors.

In the book, "Quantitative Medicine" by Mike Nichols, M.D. and Charles Davis, Ph.D., they state:

"Such activities strongly stimulate arterial repair and general heart-lung capacity. Heart attack instances plummet with such exercise, and, somewhat amazingly, cancer plummets as well. 'Intense' sounds like work, and it is. However, the time is considerably shorter. A 30-minute brisk walk, for instance, might be replaced with three 30-second sprints up a hill."

Greater benefit in less time.

Traditional Kung Fu skills training is not only loaded with short, intense exercise (which is relative to each individual), it is also composed of movements that demand high levels of coordination - which are known to develop the brain-body connection or, "neural networks" (growing new nerves!).

Keep It Moving...

Every joint must regularly move through its full range of motion and do what it was designed to do, or it will lose its full function.

Use it or lose it.

Movements that encompass this full range of motion throughout our bodies are essential for optimal health and vitality. Joints stiffen, weaken, and break down when not used. Joint replacement surgery is on the rise and doesn't have to be.

Movement is an essential component of the circulatory system as well, and the smooth flow of Qi and blood to every cell is what keeps them functioning properly.

Otherwise, disease and premature aging are certain.

Of note here is the fact that your heart wasn't meant to do all the work of moving your blood by itself. Movement, or muscle contractions, also contribute to the circulatory system. In fact, so does your breathing. It is a team effort.

———————

This Can Help You Quickly and Easily Reduce Stress and Relax Anytime, Anywhere

Place a closed fist on your belly just about an inch and a half below your navel. The thumb side of the fist is what touches your belly, so the palm of the fist hand is facing the floor or toward your feet. Place the other hand with an open palm over the fist in a way that it creates a little pressure into your belly.

Breathe through your nose. As my teacher would say, "The nose is for breathing; the mouth is for eating."

As you breathe in, you should feel the belly press out against the fist. As you breathe out your belly will naturally move in (you don't have to pull it in). Your belly should be moving in and out, not your chest.

For most people, this is difficult because for most of their lives they have been breathing improperly. This practice can change all that.

Then, working along with your heart, every breath you take will help to massage your organs as well as move the blood. Chest breathing actually works against your heart as it results in more tension in the body. This tension squeezes the vessels making the pathway smaller and increasing blood pressure.

A good way to learn and practice this is while lying down in bed or on the floor. You can even place a book over your lower abdomen and watch it rise and fall with each breath. With regular practice, you can return to this natural way of breathing all the time.

Breathing like this, the way you were meant to breathe, is also a wonderful way to relax and melt away stress.

PART THREE

Know Your "P's" And "Q's"

How To Get What You Want, and More, From the Practice

There's a saying, "The easy way is the hard way; the hard way is the easy way."

This section is all about that. You have to be willing to do the work necessary to make the kind of changes you want in your life. This practice can be a lot of fun, but you've got to do what it takes.

The following chapters dive into this further so you can get the most of the time and effort you invest.

CHAPTER 12

Find Your Special *Place*

Although modern perspectives of the martial arts from movies and pay-per-view MMA fights may have convinced the general public that it's all about fighting and violence, there's a whole other world of martial arts that sees the training as so much more. That it is deeply steeped in a tradition of teaching people how to live in this world.

How to practice is really how to live. You can look at your whole life as a practice. Don't think about punching, kicking, grappling, and blocking as all the martial arts are about. Isn't it interesting that the Chinese martial arts, although there are over 300 different styles, are known collectively as "Kung Fu"? As previously described, this term essentially means *acquired skill through consistent effort over time.*

Here we are going to discuss the 11 "P's" and a couple of "Q's" of how to practice and acquire this skill.

The First P: *Place*
The first most important thing on this list is Place.

Traditional people, native people, people living the old way such as the Bushmen in the Kalahari, the Native Americans way back when, people who live in accordance with the Dao, or the natural way, all had special teachings of the old ways that they passed down generation to generation. These old ways, the only way they knew, go back thousands upon thousands, even over a million years.

One of the most common and consistent things they teach their children is to find a place, a special place, a secret spot.

For what?

A place to *be*. That's it.

It's a place to practice. A place to be you. It's time with yourself. It's a way to find your center. It's a way to start your day from a peaceful state of mind.

You want to practice martial arts?

One thing we tell students is you've got to *show up*.

In the martial arts world, the training hall is commonly referred to as the "dojang" (or "dojo" in Japanese). However, the term refers to so much more than a "training hall" - a more recent mistranslation or simplification. It is literally a place to work on oneself - a place of enlightenment / awakening / nirvana / self-realization / heaven or whatever term you prefer. It is a place where you have the potential to raise your consciousness. It is the place where you can find your true self and enjoy more clarity in your life. It is a sanctuary, and each student's responsibility is to keep it that way.

It does not matter if you are Christian or Jew, Muslim or Hindu, Buddhist or Agnostic. It does matter that you believe what you believe and follow your own way rather than just the way you were raised or because you've been convinced by others. Your practice only strengthens your connection to your true beliefs. Only you can decide what is right for you and whether your practice is spiritual for you or not.

It is for me.

Find Your Own Special Place

It is essential to have your own place somewhere. Somewhere that feels right.

The first time you find a place, it may not be right. You go there, you try to practice and... it's just okay. It may just be the first open space you find. Some people find a driveway, a tennis court, a black top somewhere, or just an open field of grass. Someplace where they can practice.

Finding a place in nature can be much better. It can have a better feeling than some place that's been built upon. Your backyard may suffice. You have to figure that out for yourself. Does it feel right?

Once you find this special place, I recommend that you go there every day, just like the native peoples taught their children. It was a regular part of what they did and how they lived. They knew the importance of connecting with the natural world and discovering their own true nature. They understood that true courage is found in silence.

As Often as You Can

If every day is just too much for you, how about every other day? Or at least go once a week. Spend some time in nature, alone. Do your best to get to your special place regularly. Hopefully, you get in some personal time and practice there.

What kind of practice? It could be the techniques you've learned in class. The only way to master anything is through repetition.

It could be sitting and simply watching with a more outward meditation. It could be with your eyes closed, going inward with your meditation. But you give yourself that time to feel calm and centered before going into your day. Or, if it's impossible for you in the morning, go at another time of day or a couple of times a week or even once a week, but you've got to connect.

But first, you've got to find that place. And once you do you'll understand.

Wherever, Whenever

I've always had my special place where years of blood, sweat, and tears were spilled. And wherever I go, even when I go on vacation, the first thing I do once settled, is to find a place to start the day with practice and meditation.

I've practiced on beaches, on hotel roof tops, in small rooms, in the woods among the trees, parking lots, tennis courts, wherever I can and whenever I had an opportunity. Actually, I still do. Once you know what to do, you can too.

I've even meditated at Grand Central Station in NYC during rush hour (with someone looking out for me!) just to prove a point.

Is It Private?

A few years ago, when my family and I moved, there were open fields and tennis courts nearby. There was plenty of space. But the feeling was never right in that place. I'd go, I'd get in my practice, but it felt a bit more mechanical sometimes.

It's funny, because as long as I've been teaching, I've always told students, "Don't worry about people watching you. Just continue practicing and ignore them. Eventually, they'll get bored and leave." I've had this happen many times over the years. You can also look at it as a challenge for you to keep your focus since in the real world the environment is rarely perfect.

Once a woman was watching. She approached and asked, "You alright?"

People would think something was wrong with me! What's wrong with walking around in circles on a basketball court with my hands facing the pole that holds up the basket? That's where I happened to be, and that's what I was doing... for over an hour every day. What's wrong with that?

In China, it is perfectly normal to be practicing Qigong, Tai Chi, or even walking around a tree first thing in the morning. That last one may be rare, as is the art of Ba Gua Zhang, but it's still understood. They understand and respect meditation and personal quiet time. At the Temple of Heaven Park in Beijing, thousands line up at dawn to get in and do their many morning exercises.

That was one of the problems with this new place near my home. It felt like I was in a fishbowl. Early in the morning, before going to work, people would have their coffee or take their break. Midday they would park facing me and have their lunch. There was just no escape!

Whether they were or they weren't, I felt like I was their entertainment. As I mentioned, I don't generally care about people watching me, but in this location where people can park their cars facing me, it was very comfortable for them to watch me and so it was like I was on display.

Therefore, if there's parking around your spot (especially facing your practice area) or a place for people to hang out around your spot, you may not feel as peaceful.

If you can find a nice space behind some brush or trees that obstruct the view, it can feel very private and protected. I have found areas like this allow me to go deeper and get somewhat lost in my physical practice or meditation.

There may be a fence there, there may be some bushes with the fence, some ivy on the fence, whatever, but something to create some separation between you, your place, and the rest of the world.

You feel good, that way you can let go. You can practice more deeply. Finding the right place can make all the difference.

Is It Quiet and Peaceful?

If there is too much activity around you, such as people walking and talking, it may be too much of a distraction for you.

Maybe it's in the middle of a park where there is a bicycle path, or a running path, and people are talking loudly, even early in the morning.

It's nicer when all you hear are the sounds of nature. You can tune into that, and it helps you drop your thoughts and meditate.

Is It Safe?

You want to make sure it's safe. No one should be able to sneak up behind you if you are sitting in meditation. You should feel that you can remain settled there. You don't want to be overly concerned with your surroundings. You want to know that in your special place you're safe.

Are You Comfortable There? Does It *Feel* Right?

It's important that the place you choose feels right to you. This can be as simple or as difficult as you make it. Just don't put off this personal time until you find the perfect place!

I suggest you get in the habit of giving yourself some personal time alone somewhere, anywhere for the time being.

In the Meantime, Keep Looking...

You may surprise yourself with all the special places you can find if you know how to look.

Look at a map, you may be surprised what's there. You'll find blocks of open space that people rarely use. I've found blocks of wooded areas right in the middle of the busy towns I've lived in that it appeared no one knew existed.

Simply look for a green area on a map and go check it out. You never know what treasure of a special place you may find.

Maybe early in the morning, no one is there. Just take notice of the setup.

Maybe you find a special place that you only get to once a week or so because you have to drive there. So, you may go there only once a week, but you go someplace else nearby that's easy to get to daily.

Does Your Place Inspire You?

Your special place should inspire you. You'll likely find this inspiration in a place in a natural setting. Sit for a bit and experience how it comes alive. If you get a good feeling there, you'll look forward to going, Just like in our special training space, our dojang/dojo. It is a special place where students are learning more about themselves than most other endeavors. It is designed for that very purpose.

I hope you can find your own personal spot outside the dojang that gives you that kind of feeling. It should feel very special to you, even sacred.

And when you have that feeling, you look forward to getting there, consistently.

CHAPTER 13

You've Got To Be Willing To *Push* Yourself

Up the intensity and train hard!

You get to your place, you show up. You then have to push yourself. You've got to be willing to sweat. You've got to be willing to work. You're going to feel muscles burning, shaking, and aching.

We have these limitations, then if we're not working against them, nudging against our limitations, those limitations are going to become worse. What you're able to do gradually diminishes. The ceiling gets lower. For example, if you stop reaching for things with your arm, little by little, you won't be able to. It won't work. It will eventually just freeze up on you.

Your brain stops sending fluids, nutrients, and oxygen where it isn't needed, and that part of your body dries up and degenerates. Then you can't reach for anything. So if you're not taking your body through a range of motion, that range is going to get smaller and smaller.

Every time you sleep, you shrink. That's why some stretching and moving gently with various joints, gradually increasing and reaching for its normal full range, even for a few moments, is crucial to starting your day off right. Just lying in bed for the night your body gets used to the lack of movement. So we've got to push ourselves first thing in the morning and start loosening up a little bit. It's a far more effective approach than coffee!

Do you sit a lot at work? Take a look at your posture, the position you're in most of the day. If you spend all day sitting, your legs are bent so the back of your legs, your hamstrings, are going to get shorter. Your back and hips are also going to get tight and not work properly. With your body weight crushing your buttocks while you sit, how much blood flow do you think reaches the area?

Are your hips and tailbone tucked under and forward so your lower back is rounded? Then you wonder why there's so many back problems, knee problems, hip problems and sciatica.

Then there is the time you most likely spend with your head forward, as you lean into the computer monitor or frequently look down as you text or use your smart phone. This leads to all sorts of neck problems and maybe even headaches.

You really do have to get over yourself!

I was referring to your posture. :)

It's not just "Father Time." It's your body changing over time according to with what you do regularly.

How hard can we push? What's too much? What's not enough?

Let's take a quick detour to look at the Q's...

CHAPTER 14

The "Q's": *Quality* and *Quantity*

There are two ways to look at quality vs. quantity.

First off, if it's real skill you're after, repetition is the mother of skill. You can't expect to run through all sorts of different drills "just to remember" and ever develop any real skills.

This is why martial arts that test or grade based on the number of skills, sequences, or techniques the student can remember is killing the quality of their martial art. More is actually less.

The most effective approach is to work diligently and consistently on specific skills, drills, or techniques until mastered before moving on to anything new. Develop a depth to your skills and understanding of the practical use rather than spreading it out thinly and superficially. Quality over quantity.

And it's the basics that make the master.

I was once at a large martial arts industry event with teachers and school owners in attendance from all over the country and even some from outside of the U.S. One class was joint-locking related, and my partner was bragging to me about the 573 joint-locking techniques in his system. He clearly wanted me to know how accomplished he was.

Then some simple joint locks were shared by the instructor of the class and my partner struggled with them to the point of frustration. Enough said.

Secondly...

If it's physical training, what's too much?

When the quality of the training suffers, meaning you start getting sloppy or have less control of the movements, back off. It's not how much you do, it's how much you can do correctly that counts the most. If you train sloppiness, your skills will be just that: sloppy.

You also risk injury when you get sloppy. If you find yourself regularly getting injured every time you ramp it up and get serious you're either over doing it, or you're doing something wrong. You may simply have poor body mechanics that should be evaluated and corrected by an expert (who may or may not be your teacher - it all depends on how well trained he or she is in biomechanics or human movement).

Also, when you're too exhausted to do your normal day-to-day tasks, and you don't feel good, you're doing too much. Now you've got to look at both ends of that. You could be doing too much physically, or you may not be getting enough rest or enough sleep to balance that activity. Maybe it's a nutritional deficiency.

But that is pushing yourself: we have to push. In life, we have to push. Is it ever enough? When is it too much?

When your tank is 100% full, you're well rested, you've eaten, etc., but you're spending more than 100% where does that leave you?

If you have $100 dollars in the bank, try to write a $150 check. Not only does it bounce, it costs you more, doesn't it? That's exactly how your body works. This deficit is going to start taxing your "Original Qi", "Essence", or "*Jing*", (精), according to Chinese medicine. It's a lot like the internal battery you were born with. You tax your body; the charge comes down even faster. You age faster. The deficit multiplies.

You can think of your Jing as the battery in your car. It has a limited life. It needs to be regularly recharged. As it ages, it loses power and gradually fully charges less and less. If you abuse it and leave your lights on long enough when you park at the mall, there's a good chance you won't have enough juice to get it started when you want to leave.

So how do you know what is too much?

You have to go by how you feel. Keep pushing and pushing and overdo it, and you're going to get pushed back. You may get knocked down with various illnesses, sometimes even a serious one.

You may be thinking, "I can't stop! You don't understand!"

I would say, "What if you broke your leg? What if you get sick?" How many times in your life have you seen someone like that? Doesn't know how to stop, keeps going, going, going, and all of a sudden, they've got cancer. All of a sudden, all those things that they thought they had to go for, push for, are not so important anymore. Their perspective can change very quickly.

What's too much? What's not enough? Can you tell when you're lazy? Can you tell when you've overdone it? Remember: quality over quantity.

So you get to your special place, and you're practicing. How do you feel when you leave? You should feel a little proud of yourself. You come to class, you train, you go home. You got in, you worked hard, you're tired. But you feel good about yourself.

Real Confidence

This is where real confidence comes from. You start to believe in yourself. You're actually doing it. But if you're a little lazy, frequently missing class, or not getting to your special place, not practicing regularly, you won't feel so good about yourself. You know you're not pushing hard enough. Or you go to your spot, you're there two hours, but you're so-so with your efforts with a lot of the time wasted. How good was that practice?

Some might get together with a training partner. They mean well, but then 90% of the time is talking. You got out there first thing in the morning, spent two hours together, but what was the level of quality for that practice?

That's the thing, so many people talk about having time constraints but how much time is wasted? We all have 24 hours. Some get more out of it than others and, therefore, have a lot more to show for it.

Our bodies respond to the demand or lack of demand we put on them. It will grow and get stronger or atrophy and get weaker depending on your day-to-day efforts.

It's up to you.

Now back to the P's:

If you want to get the most out of the time you can devote to your practice, you must be fully *Present*...

CHAPTER 15

Be Fully *Present* With Laser-Sharp Focus

How can you do anything right if you're not present? Being present means concentration. Being present means focus. I must be focused on what I'm doing in this moment. Two people get together to practice, and they're talking back and forth. This is not about practice anymore. What was your purpose in being there? Are you getting as much out of it as you can? Only if you're focused.

You go to work, same thing. If you're an employer, how efficient are your employees? How many coffee breaks? How much talking around the water cooler time? How much gossip is going around? Most studies say we barely get in two hours of real, efficient work out of an eight-hour day. Millions and millions of dollars wasted even when people are working hard and pushing themselves, but they're not efficient. They're not productive. What a waste of time. You feel like you're working hard but little gets done.

It seems to me that more productive work would result in the higher wages most employees want. Working hard isn't enough.

When you're fully present, you do better. You make fewer mistakes, so you don't have to fix things as often. When you get it done right the first time, you can move on to whatever is next.

Being present can change everything about your life. Imagine only working two efficient hours and getting the same productivity that most people get in eight? You could get twice as much done in half the time and have the rest of the day off! (And there are people who work for themselves who are able to do just that. They are very efficient as well as productive).

Unfortunately, it doesn't work that way for most people, does it? Get more done then more is expected, isn't it? It sure would be nice if we could change all that as a society.

It does raise a good argument for figuring out how to work for yourself, though, doesn't it? But that's a different book.

If being present is being focused, what should you focus on? Let's answer this with a martial arts practice. Do you need more strength? Do you need more flexibility? Are you feeling a little stiff? Where specifically? How's your conditioning? Are you quickly out of breath? Could your coordination be improved? As a martial artist, can you generate effective power in your techniques?

So, what is it you need to focus on? Do you know?

It can be any specific part of your practice. Let's say for now it's the hands. Or your body. Or footwork. What else do we have? Breath. Concentration. Application. Accuracy. I like to say what we're doing is, "BodyMind Training™." Remember that: BodyMind Training™, using the body to train the mind. There is no separation between the body and the mind. It only seems so due to where you place your attention.

There are many ways to do BodyMind Training™. How are the traditional martial arts different? One way is that the movements have meaning.

Dancers can be phenomenal. They'll demonstrate amazing coordination, agility, flexibility, strength, and beauty. They have to concentrate, but the concentration is not the same as in the traditional martial arts. When I move my hand, I have a clear reason. Is it for defense? Is it for attack? If it is for attack, where? When? What opportunity is available now? What do I see?

If it's more for health, or the Qigong side, the work is on coordinating breath with focus and movement. When you're moving through different postures, what do you feel? What are you trying to do?

For example, you might imagine you're pushing a mountain. That connects your body and mind with intention.

When you're absolutely present in that practice, the benefits skyrocket. It's very different. My teacher always said, "20 minutes with focus is better than 2 hours without."

We have to be fully present if we want the most results. Very few have extra time these days. You need to get very efficient with what time you have. Without focus, you're wasting time.

If you have time to waste, that's fine. I don't. If you're like me, you need a purpose. You need a reason, you need to know what you're trying to accomplish so that when you get to your *place,* you can *push* in the most productive way. That's what proper practice is about.

People often say, "Practice makes perfect." This isn't true. Practice makes permanent. And poor practice makes bad habits that can be very hard to break.

Think about that in your life. You smoke, you know it causes lung cancer. You may have even known people who have died from lung cancer, but you still don't stop.

Sure, there's a chemical addiction involved with nicotine, but if you want health, *you're practicing more for illness.* You've made a habit for illness. You don't really want health then, do you? Based on your actions, the smoking is more important to you than your health.

Being present is being aware of what you do.

You want a good relationship? You have to pay attention to the other person. You have to know what their needs are, their wants, their desires. You have to know when the things you do rub them wrong. And you can't get mad at them if they don't know what rubs you the wrong way. Your job is you!

Do you get angry with them because they don't do what you think they should do? This is a waste of energy and a bad habit that is never going to bring peace or an improved relationship. You can't "fix" them. You only can fix (change) yourself.

Being present teaches you that. If you're present, you can realize what you're doing, how you're reacting, what you're neglecting, what you're not doing as well as you could or should. That you can fix, if you so desire.

If you learn something that you find beneficial in some way and you want your partner to learn the same, remember: they're not you. Let them figure it out on their own, when they're ready, and in their own way.

Maybe you do certain things that make them happier, then they naturally try to make you happier as well. That's being present. You live mindfully with awareness of what you do. Focus is in the moment. With too many distractions it's very difficult to be present.

But don't get upset again if they don't immediately respond to your efforts! (and thinking, "See, nothing works!")

Are you aware of what you do in your free time? All the in-between? How much time is wasted? Do you frequently do things "just to pass the time?" Time is your life. How much do you want to waste?

It's one thing to get up early, get to your place, push yourself hard, sweat, and feel good. Then, what about all the in-between time? What do you fill your head with? Is it constant trash on television? Or maybe a certain kind of music that's got a real negative message. It's all creating habits, or just noise because you have to have distraction. You don't like quiet.

But everything you expose yourself to on a regular basis is having an effect on you (including talk shows, music lyrics, your conversations, etc.) Is it what you want? Is it making your life better somehow?

Just this morning my daughter had the TV on, she was watching a movie. The movie ended and it's a DVD, so it just kept repeating forever and ever, so I turned it off. She came running in, screaming that she was watching that, while she was in the other room. That's pretty interesting. How do you do that? She just liked the music. She liked that sound. Of course, this was fine, even wonderful. That makes her happy.

I have nothing against music. That would be ridiculous as it brings so many so much joy. However, what I am talking about is having the presence of mind to realize that we don't like it when it's quiet. This is a problem.

We want something other than silence because the peace isn't there. We make these choices, and we have these habits that we're not aware of, and each has positive or negative effects on our ability to be present.

That's why people find it so difficult to meditate. That's why Blaise Pascal once said, "All the troubles of the world stem from a man's inability to sit quietly in a room alone."

CHAPTER 16

Some Things Take Time: You've Got To Have *Patience*

Things take time. In due time, whatever it is you're searching for, hoping for, desiring, it may come. Lack of patience comes from attachment. You cannot practice with a focus on results. You'll most likely get upset when you don't reach them. It's one thing to set a goal, and I think we all should, but a goal cannot be rigid. A goal is only to give you direction. "I want to be good at footwork." Okay, so you make a program practicing footwork.

"I want to be stronger." So you make a program for strength. That's a goal. But how long it actually takes you to reach your goal, I don't know. You don't know. You can't make a plan that you're going to be a master by a certain date. It may help to motivate you, but it doesn't work like that.

"I will be a black belt by June 11, 2019." This is crazy stuff. You have no idea how you're going to develop.

Over the years, we've received numerous calls where someone has asked, "How long does it take to get a black belt?" I have no idea. It takes how long it takes. Everyone is different.

And it's not the point of the practice. Not by a long shot.

Other times, we want something now, and if we had just waited and been more patient, it would have been better. Something better comes along. But because we're impatient, many times we don't really get what we want. This is a habit, too.

"Be not afraid of growing slowly. Be afraid of standing still."
- Chinese proverb

It Takes How Long It Takes

It doesn't matter how eager or impatient you are about something. If you plant a tree in hopes of enjoying the shade or the beauty, it's growth requires nourishment, sunshine, *and time*. When it sprouts, it takes how long it takes to grow to maturity and its full size. If you attempt to hurry it along with your impatience and pull on that sprout to try and make it grow faster... you will kill it.

What if we just go with the flow a little more?
Stay the course and let things work themselves out.
Work down the list:

- Go to my special place every day.
- Push myself and train hard. Do my thing.
- Be aware. Be fully engaged and focused on what I'm doing.

Then let the chips fall as they may in my practice and in my life. Accept what is, knowing I've done all I can.

If I'm living in a way with a direction in mind, and I stay on that road based on the little things that are actually the most important things, I feel good. I'm happy. I'm at peace.

What more do you want? What end point do you have to get to?

Just stay the course with consistent effort over time, and you will get where that road goes. It's inevitable.

How many times have we heard of the gold medalist who's trained their whole life since they were a child, and they win the gold medal, and that's it. Or the entertainer? Hollywood star? They're on the top of the top, they reached the peak. Now what? What's next? Many become lost after reaching the top or experiencing their one defining moment. It's all downhill from there.

How many have you read about who became drug addicts? Multiple divorces? In trouble with the law? They fall off that top. They reached the top that most think is so great. All the money and partying, and all the great stuff, and yet... they're miserable.

The destination only gives direction. It's the journey that matters most. Patience is all about the journey.

And when you talk about the journey you can't leave out Perseverance...

CHAPTER 17

Perseverance:

You Only Fail When You Quit

I like this road, but I keep getting knocked off. So many obstacles! Okay, get back on, try again. Go around, try again. Whatever it takes; if it's important enough to you.

Once we had wasps who made their home just outside our back doorway. Oh boy, were they thick-headed! I don't like to spray chemicals and kill them off. Instead, I threw water and broke up the hive they were building.

Let me tell you something, for weeks, they kept coming back. I'd break it down, and they'd build it again. I'd break it down, and they'd come back and build it again... and again... and again.

Every time I knocked them down, they got up. I knocked them down again, they got up again. Seemed like if I knocked them down a thousand times, they would get up a thousand and one.

Then one day I sat down outside of my doorway and spoke to them. I said, "Do you know there's a lot of other places you could go and build your home? There are lots of woods over there." Believe it or not, a couple of days later they left, finally.

Was it because of what I said? I don't know, but it was amazing. All of a sudden, they found another place.

Fall down a thousand times, get up a thousand and one. Life is going to knock you down, you've got to find a way to get back up and keep going forward.

You go to your place, you don't go to your place - one day, you just can't get there. What do you do the next day? Make a habit not to go? You get back there again, if you're serious about the road you chose to take.

Perseverance has a lot to do with developing your will. The will to keep going. The will to do what you're supposed to do even when you don't feel like it. You know, you don't feel like practicing. You don't feel like going to class. You don't feel like working on that project you're supposed to at work.

Perseverance is doing it anyway.

You don't feel like it? Do it anyway. Get started anyway.

Strikeout King

If you read about successful people, you will frequently find that they had more failures than most.

Did you know that Babe Ruth was once known as "The King of Strikeouts?" How could this be? Because he was always swinging for the fences.

It's an interesting story. The Babe was considered the greatest baseball player that ever lived. Did he strike out a few times and declare, "I'm done with this!"? Of course not! That's how he became so great. He had no fear of failure. He knew that people came to the ballpark to see him hit home runs, so that's what he went for every time.

Dedicated to Greatness

Then there's the story of Michael Jordan getting cut from the varsity basketball team when he was a sophomore in high school. As I understand it, he was only 5'11" back then, and the varsity coach chose another sophomore instead, who was a friend of Jordan's, because he was 6'7".

Jordan has told this story countless times, including how he went home and cried in his room after reading the team roster, but the key here is how it drove him to the greatness he is known for. It did not crush him. He became *obsessed*.

Steve Jobs was called obsessed because he wanted to create nothing short of perfection and ultimately change the world with technology.

Please, no offense meant to those with a disorder, but it's been said, "Obsessed is just a word the lazy use to describe the dedicated." To become great, you can expect lazy people to call you obsessed, while they sit on the couch, remote in hand...

Unemployed? You must be dedicated to finding a job. Go for a job, don't get it. Go for another job. Still don't get it. What are you going to do? Give up and go live in the street?

Perseverance Is the Only Way

You've got to keep going... next... next... Salesmen have to knock on door after door after door. They will never have success if they don't know how to knock on the door, get kicked in the teeth, and go to the next door, as if nothing happened while maintaining a positive attitude. If not, there is a nice cold curb to sleep on. No matter how many times, just go again. No matter what, just shake it off and step up...

Shake It Off and Step Up

There was once an old donkey that fell into a well. He cried and cried, but there was nothing anyone could do. The farmer who owned the donkey decided that rather than allow him to keep suffering, he would simply bury him there, since he was old and the well was dry, and he was planning to fill it in anyway.

The farmer got some help from his family and friends to fill in the well. They all grabbed shovels and got to work. Dirt quickly began to cover the donkey, who was now wailing loudly as he realized what was going on.

However, it wasn't long before he quieted down.

Thinking it odd, and wondering how the donkey could become quiet so quickly, the farmer told everyone to stop for a moment so he could look down and see what happened. He was pleasantly surprised by what he saw.

When the shovelfuls of dirt started piling up on and around him, the donkey began to shake the dirt off his back and step up on the now rising pile of dirt.

So the farmer and his help continued, and the donkey did too. Every new shovelful prompted him to shake it off and step up, shake it off and step up... until eventually and amazingly, he stepped right up and out of the well! So the next time you feel like life just keeps piling more and more trouble, difficulty, and rejection on top of you, remember the donkey: just shake it off and step up!

There's another "P" that comes to mind here. As I've repeated a few times, you have to get to your place in order to push yourself and when you're pushing you've got to maintain focus, and no matter how much you focus or how hard you push, you can't be in a rush, you need to have patience.

And when you don't get what you want, when you want it, you've got to keep going anyway. But what will help you to keep going? Having *Passion*...

CHAPTER 18

Passion: The Fire Within

Think about a time when you just got something you really, really wanted.

How about that first date with someone you really liked? Can you remember after that first date how life went? Weren't you in a great mood? Did anyone ask, "What's with you?"

How about those of you who received that letter of acceptance from the college you wanted so badly to attend?

Or you got the return call letting you know how well your interview went and that you got the job you were trying so hard to get?

Do you remember how you felt? And how energized did it make you feel?

You were passionate about these things and from within you were jolted into all that extra energy for you to use in your life.

How do you develop such an on-going passion for something?

It goes back to who or what you listen to (people, music, etc.), what you watch on TV, and what you're reading. Do you read stories that inspire you to choose and stay on a better more fulfilling path (or to stay and persevere on the road you're on if you like where it's headed)? Or do you just spend your down time with entertainment that really doesn't serve any purpose for you other than distracting you from "the real world?"

Movies, TV, etc... time goes by. How did it serve you? Sure, we all need entertainment. We all need fun. We don't want to be overly rigid through our lives, but there are numerous books, videos and even courses that you can take to make good use of your time, so you learn and grow. Then your life can evolve rather than being the same every day as you just get older and life gets harder.

Go to a bookstore and see if something just catches your eye. Maybe something about peaceful living. Feed your brain some new ways of thinking. Hopefully this book you're reading is doing some of that.

Only you know what does it for you, but at least you're feeding yourself information to start developing passion because the more passion you have for something, whatever that is, your relationship, your work, your practice, the more energy you will have to pursue your dreams and the less outside motivation you will need.

It's not as hard to get up when you're excited about it. When you don't have a reason, it can start to become a burden, grudgingly going to practice thinking, "I know this is good for me, so I'm going..." begrudgingly.

That attitude is going to weaken you. It's going to drain you. Everything you do with that attitude spends more energy than it should. And life gets hard.

Why is an advanced martial artist, someone who has the skills and has been practicing a long time, able to push themselves so much harder for so much longer?

Think about that.

The beginner has to work on just doing this right, doing that right, trying to follow and figure things out, but the advanced person already has developed the habits. They already know the movements more reflexively. It's now more natural for them, so they spend less energy yet have a better quality of practice.

It's like the first time you went to a job that's brand new. You're nervous, you're unsure. You're trying to learn everything, and you want to look good at the same time. But once you've been there for a while, it becomes second nature.

If you've got a training program all set up and you go out to your practice place already knowing what you're going to do, you don't need to think about it. You just do it. And when you have a goal in mind with your practice, you just have to follow the program. You just have to see it through.

Then, because you know the movements, what's happening now?

Expanding Your Consciousness

Your practice can go from the most simplified to more and more complex. And when that happens, you naturally start to expand your consciousness. You'll start to notice your presence increasing without effort. You start to be more aware of the things you do without trying.

It's very interesting how your practice and your life will parallel. As your skills improve through *BodyMind Training*™ like this, it's a natural consequence in your life to be happier, more peaceful, more present. Your friends, your family, the people you work with will notice you're different. I can't tell you over the years how many students told me this.

I read the things students say in the lessons they complete. These are the things that come out. Something is happening as a consequence of the positive influence. That's why reading before you go to sleep, for 5, 10, or 15 minutes, is feeding yourself things that help you to practice and to build the passion, which results in it positively affecting your life.

When you're doing the work, and you're getting results, you're more excited. You have more energy. Think about it. You come home at the end of the day, and you're tired. You had all your work and other responsibilities to complete. You don't want to be bothered, and you sit there, and then somebody rings the front bell.

"Who's that?" you don't even want to get out of your chair.

If they said, "You won the lottery!" do you think you could muster up some energy?

If you have passion, if you have the energy to get the work done, to get out there and do what it takes, you'll enjoy what you're doing. In other words, having passion for your job, for the work you do, leads to a more productive and rewarding work life. Having passion for the relationship you're in leads to a better and more enjoyable love life.

If you have the passion, you will have the energy to do what needs to be done. You'll *want* to do it.

If we're not excited, life is hard. Isn't life hard enough already?

Once the passion is found, then we just need clear direction, so we don't waste our efforts and spend our limited energy fruitlessly.

You can be excited just running around in circles (and I'm not talking about Ba Gua "circle-walking" here). I mean living in the chaos, but with direction.

And that's why next up is *Purpose*...

CHAPTER 19

Spark The Fire With *Purpose*

Passion comes from having a reason... your purpose. Why you do what you do.

Can you see the future? If you have a vision for your life, it gives you direction. Then you know why you're making such an effort. Now you have your purpose.

What's your purpose? What's going to give you that passion? Is your training driven by the ability to exercise in a more interesting way? Is health your main motivation? Or is it self defense?

You want to feel safe walking the streets. You want to know you can protect yourself and you're driven by that. Maybe you had a bad experience that left you feeling vulnerable, and you never want to feel like that again. You want to feel empowered.

Most people come to martial arts for one of those two reasons: they're bored with the gym and want a more interesting way to get in great shape, or they want to feel more confident, and believe that knowing how to defend themselves will do that for them.

However, could the purpose be you simply enjoy it? If you do something for the love of it, you just feel good. You just feel better when you're doing it.

Although I may have started with self defense in mind, as have many of my students, we have kept at it for so long because of so much more.

Our experience of this practice is more happiness and fulfillment. You can feel more at peace, and you don't need a lofty goal to reach.

Does your purpose have to be a goal? No, I don't believe so.

You may have heard that it's the journey that matters most and not the destination. However, don't forget: it's the destination that gives direction.

A goal is something that gives you direction. You have to know what road to get on in order to get where you'd like to go.

However, you can always change that direction. You might say you really want that goal but you keep falling off the path and you may or may not get back to it. That's why this book also had a section on perseverance.

You fall down, you get back up. Fall off the horse, get back on. But sometimes the goal changes because you discover you don't want it as much as you thought you did. Or, maybe your understanding changes.

Some people get confused about that purpose. And if you don't have that purpose, if you don't have a good reason for why you're doing what you're doing, the passion can diminish. The driving force within can deflate. You can start to lose that drive and be easily swayed off course, especially when it gets too hard.

So it's very important that you have some reason why you're doing what you're doing.

Even if you have what many would consider the lower end of the spectrum of desirable jobs (I'll leave that up to you!), your passion can be how it's a stepping stone to bigger and better things. Or, it pays the rent or mortgage and puts food in your children's bellies so you're grateful and you just want to be the best at what you do, regardless.

There's a story about how people lose it on an assembly line. They're doing the same thing over and over, day in and day out, so they feel like they're losing their mind. But one worker, in particular, was all smiles as every day he tried to break records from his previous days.

He would work on getting faster or more efficient and every day was a new challenge. He created a purpose for every day he was at the same job where the others were complaining and losing their minds.

We can do that with anything. Any purpose serves its purpose.

If you don't have a reason why you do what you do, it's a lot harder to keep it up. Your reason could simply be, "I feel better doing it. I'm happier, healthier, more productive, and more focused." Is that reason enough? I think so. Just take notice of these things because sometimes we forget.

Doing your best can be a purpose. Knowing this, that you gave your all, allows you to move forward in spite of results, with a *Passive* attitude...

CHAPTER 20

Lighten Up! The *Passive* Attitude

When someone is learning meditation, I tell them it's very important to keep a passive attitude. It's no different with your physical practice. Keep a passive attitude. Does that apply in our work or in our relationships?

"I don't care." Is that what a passive attitude is? "Whatever."

How can I tell you to have passion and then be passive? Isn't this conflicting advice?

Being passive as I mean it is about being non-judgmental and unattached to results. Our attachment to results, our believing things should be a certain way, is what creates most of our suffering. We want things the way we want them. And we want them that way *now*. That's why we need to be passive because then we recognize we can't control those things.

So, be passive about results. Practice just to practice.

Practice just to practice? What does that mean? The same as when I was describing that your purpose could be 'When I practice I feel better. I'm happier. I'm healthier. I'm more at peace. I'm more focused. I want more health. I want to be able to defend myself. I want all these things but..."

If you practice just to practice and you practice right, results are automatic.

Results are automatic, so there's no need to be concerned with the results. Simply do the best you can all the time. Enjoy the process.

But expecting certain results within a certain time period is a problem. There is no use looking at someone else in class who's farther along than you, but they started the same time as you, maybe even after you.

"Why are they moving along in rank and I'm not?"

How does that help you? It doesn't. That's not passive. Do the work, do it well, do it right, and you'll get there when you get there. You just aren't *there* yet. You're *here*, wherever that is. Accept it, and do what needs to be done to continue progressing. There is no other way.

Siddhartha's Secret

Have your read the book *Siddhartha* by Herman Hesse? I highly recommend it. Throughout the many challenges Siddhartha faced, he would always remember and say these three things to himself, "I can think; I can wait; I can fast."

This is similar to the military adage, "Keep calm and carry on." If you can maintain a passive attitude, being unattached and not letting your emotions get the best of you, you will be better able to think your way through any problem you face.

You can be patient knowing *some things take time*. Any lack of patience on your part isn't going to make it happen any faster. It's just going to get you unsettled and unable to perform your best at any task necessary.

And you know how people are about eating. However, if you've ever experienced fasting, you have learned you can go quite some time without food. I've gone five days myself. So, "I can fast" refers to not being needy, desperate to get what you want right now. You do your very best and let the chips fall as they may with a full understanding of what is in your power to control and what is not.

This is exactly what approaching things with a passive attitude means. Whether it's progress in your martial arts practice, in your job or career, or in finding that special someone to share your life with. It takes how long it takes and wasting all that mental and emotional energy on what you have no control over is not only not helping, it's holding you back.

How can you possibly be fully engaged in the process of doing whatever it takes to get what you want if so much of you is caught up in what you don't have?

We don't all live the same lives. We don't all think the same ways. We don't all have the same coordination or background. I even had a student who said he never kicked a ball in his life, even as a kid growing up (so using that analogy for a specific kicking technique didn't help him at all).

There are so many ways we're different. Accept yourself as you are and do all you can to continue to learn and grow. Regardless of the results, you can still feel great about yourself knowing you're doing all you can.

There is no resting on your laurels and staying the same. Everything is either growing or dying. Which do you prefer?

If you are choosing to grow, it's much easier to maintain a passive attitude, and make progress, if you have a *Plan*...

CHAPTER 21

Decide What You Want -
Make A *Plan* -
Stop Thinking

I t's a lot easier to remain passive about results when you take thought out of the equation.

But how do you do that?

At least every weekday most people have a pretty set schedule. You have work. You have home maintenance and other responsibilities. Maybe you have children to care for (and play with!)

You have a set time to get up. In fact, you most likely have an alarm go off to make sure of it.

Then comes the routine: you go to the bathroom, brush your teeth, take your shower, shave, make your breakfast (or pick something up on the way to work or school), drink your coffee (which may also be on a preset timer), etc., etc., concluding with arriving at work (or school) after a mindless drive that you don't even remember because you take the exact same route every time (while listening to some form of entertainment).

Sound familiar? How much thought do you have to put into the things you do repeatedly every day?

And who made this schedule?

At the interview to get the job you have did they tell you to make your own hours? Not likely. Most people are told when to be where and what to do when they get there.

And that's the secret to training automation.

Training Automation

Just like you have to answer to bosses, superiors, spouses, etc., how about listening to the part of you who wants something more? You know, the person who thinks it would be great to learn martial arts. Like I frequently say to students: "You each have your own personal reasons for being here. How are you going to get what you came for?"

First, you have to make a decision. Part of that decision was to find a good school and teacher. Did that? Okay, next.

Once enrolled (in a martial arts school or any other endeavor for education, career advancement, or personal growth of some sort), you then have some sort of curriculum to learn.

And each item or component of that curriculum will take some time and effort to be absorbed and for you to become comfortable, and eventually skilled with.

Most people in the martial art only train when they are at their dojang/dojo. But those who excel also put in some extra time on their own.

Not sure what to do on your own?

It's one thing to just go ahead and do your reps for kicks or punches or stances, etc. It all needs some work to get comfortable with.

However, what are you struggling with most?

It could be a skill or technique or drill of some sort. Or maybe you have some form of old injury, weakness somewhere, lack of flexibility or problems with your balance.

Whatever it is you want or need to work on, you make a decision and then, you make a plan.

Instead of shying away from the things that give you trouble (because it frustrates you or hurts your feelings or doesn't make you feel good about yourself), make a plan to work on it.

For how long?

I have no idea. It takes how long it takes.

Though my Shifu once said that when you learn something new practice it every day for one hundred days. Then, he said, "You got it."

Book Yourself

Now all you have to do is follow your plan. "Ten minutes of loosening up first thing in the morning on Mondays, Wednesdays, and Fridays" or "Every Tuesday and Friday I work on footwork for 20 minutes" or whatever you can fit in your schedule.

You have to make it as important as all your other responsibilities. For example, "On Saturdays at 8AM, it's just what I do."

If you do this, and stop arguing with yourself with things like "I'm too tired today," "I don't feel like it," "I'm never going to get it," or whatever else comes to mind, then progress is inevitable.

You already decided what you want. You made your plan. Now, stop thinking, and just do it.

(Sorry, Nike. I seriously doubt you were the first to use that phrase.)

Now keep doing it just like you do everything else that you're committed to in your schedule - without thinking and rethinking about it.

Practice Right

Your mind should be focused on the practice, as you do your very best to perform every rep of every skill, exercise, or technique as correctly as you know how.

Repeatedly doing something wrong can lead not only to bad habits that can be very hard to break, but also to injury.

Don't worry, as you consistently show up for class you should also be getting the correction you need. Be grateful (not insulted or put down in any way!) and do your best to remember and apply any corrections you receive.

It Might Hurt

At the beginning of following through your plan, you can expect at least some discomfort, especially if you're a beginner. You're asking your body to do things it hasn't done before. Just like going to the gym and lifting weights for the first time (or the first time in a while) you can get very sore!

Believe me, there are going to be plenty of times like this if you're working hard! You just have to stick to the plan anyway. The soreness will subside as your body gets more used to what you're asking of it.

And that's what makes us stronger.

Then, maybe three months or so down the road (about a hundred days, as stated above) after consistently keeping your plan (and your word to yourself), you can bring thought back into the process and evaluate how it's going.

Then, it's time to decide - should you continue the same or make a change?

To Review:

Make a decision.

Create a plan.

Then, *stop thinking and do it.*

Just like you do so many other things in your life, except this will be with intention – heading in the direction you want.

Remember, *practice just to practice*. Let progress take care of itself.

That's training automation.

Benjamin Franklin once said, "If you fail to plan you plan to fail."

I do believe he was referring to any pursuit in life.

Now let's move on to making *Progress* automatic...

CHAPTER 22

How To Make *Progress* Automatic

I've said it a few times now, practice just to practice. Here I want to discuss progress from a different angle.

We're all human. Beyond that, I don't know. So there's no reason to look beyond yourself when you're looking to progress. That's where sincerity comes in, too. You have to be honest about your efforts, your consistent efforts, over time. Why you're moving along or not.

Passive and with purpose. It is an interesting pair that may seem contradictory.

Progress, how do we measure it? How do we measure if we're making progress? Is it the color of the belt or sash around your waist?

Think a Little Deeper.

Are you happier? Are you more at peace? Do you feel better? Is your life better, somehow, because you practice?

Combine these things a little bit. Think about your reason to work. What's your attitude toward that?

"Oh, it's just how I make money. Got to pay my bills." That's it? That's your purpose at work? That's your reason for doing that job? Some people's purpose could be the challenge, the experience of doing that kind of work.

Remember the example of the person on an assembly line that was discussed in the chapter on Purpose? He made every day a new challenge even with such repetitive work.

"A way to express myself and to be creative." Well, that's the interesting thing about progress. If something is challenging in that it moves from simple to more complex things, every new level of learning will usually feel just like with anything else that is new - awkward. But keep at it and eventually, like everything else you've learned, it will become comfortable.

Maybe in a month, maybe in six, maybe in a year or more it stops feeling awkward. But when it was new it seemed so complicated.

Learning martial arts has to start out with simple things. However, for the beginner, it is still complicated because it is new. This is no different than the first time you're on a new job. First dates in a relationship. It's awkward when you're not sure yet how you should act or what you should do.

"Am I doing the right thing? Should I call now? Not call now?" All these questions we ask ourselves. How do we make progress? How do we even see the progress? How do we recognize it?

Soon you become more comfortable, and as you become more comfortable, what used to seem so complicated now seems so simple. Now you're ready for something more difficult or complex. And in time, that too will become simple once you put in the required time and effort.

That's progress.

But then, guess what? Another level to build upon for something newer, more difficult and complex.

You may start wondering again, "Am I ever going to get this?"

In a sophisticated martial art like Ba Gua Zhang, this is a never-ending process (trust me). It continues to become more and more complex, challenging your mind and your body with more complexity both externally, with technique and internally, with better and better structural integrity.

The more the complex becomes simple, the more developed you have become. Even while in a seemingly chaotic situation, you will remain calmer, more focused and in control. Everything can *seem slower to you.*

In time, your creative abilities begin to shine through. Once the principles become ingrained in your understanding the future of the art for you becomes unlimited. Just as it goes in the Daoist view of the universe and its creation:

- Dao Creates One
- One Creates Two
- Two Create Three
- Three Create All Things

And yet, it is all Dao. The ultimate complexity must never lose its center; its root. We must never lose our root or true nature.

With a clear understanding of the principles, you can make it your own, with infinite possibilities.

Making it your own. Think about that. It's the ultimate goal: To internalize the principles of Dao while living in this crazy, wonderful world.

But how easily do we fall into a pattern and then just mindlessly do the same thing over and over, making no progress at all?

"But, Shifu, you're supposed to do repetition, right?"

Yes, of course! But never mindlessly. Always maintain purpose. Stay centered and focused regardless of the complexity. Don't just copy. Learn to create.

I'm not just talking martial arts - work, play, relationships. Do you just get into a rut where it's the same thing over and over, to where you're just comfortable in the pattern, and you don't want to change?

How do you make progress? How do you make progress in your professional life? How do you make progress in your personal life? Can you really just stay the same?

Nothing stays the same. That is a principle in this world. Change is a principle. Ba Gua Zhang is also called, *"the art of change."*

"Ba Gua" is the principle of change. Nothing in this world stays the same. That is a natural law. So why are we so unnatural, wanting things to be one way? We can get stuck in our ways, making it impossible because we're comfortable. What's comfortable? What's satisfied?

Pride.

We want to feel good about ourselves. We want to look good to others. People have killed over "losing face."

We want success in everything we do and giving up prematurely due to difficulties or not feeling successful soon enough is why so many never reach their true potential or their dreams. Progress stalls.

Change is difficult. It can be uncomfortable. You may feel out of sorts and not yourself for a while. But that's how you grow.

Don't let *Pride* hold you back.

CHAPTER 23

Humility Wins; *Pride* Loses

Pride in the martial arts is thinking, "I'm good! I'm so good. I'm better than everybody. I can beat up whoever I want. When I walk into a room, it's good to know I can kick everybody's ass."

So sad.

That's not how a martial artist thinks. That's how a bully thinks.

Some people practice two or three years, make good progress, and then think they're good and that's it. They may stick around for years and never progress again. They learn more techniques, but their skill level never changes.

They got comfortable with their level. They don't like that awkward feeling of not being good at something, so they just remember, and they move on. They're a little better than the beginner at remembering because they have the first two, three, four years of progress and growth, but that's it. That's it for their development.

Are You Teachable?

Allowing that awkward feeling, accepting what is true about your current level of skill and being passive in your attitude toward it is the only way to make real progress. Then you can focus on the training and getting better, rather than on what you can't do so well, yet.

Never be satisfied. Be happy when someone with more time, knowledge and experience than you offers their help. Get excited when you get corrected or discover what you're not so good at. Why take it as a personal attack? Now you know what to focus on.

Pride puts a monkey wrench in progress. Don't let your ego get in the way of mastery.

As soon as you're satisfied, as soon as you're comfortable, progress stops.

It Can Happen to Anything in Your Life

Your martial arts practice can die when you get too comfortable. Your job might die too, or you'll just be bored out of your mind if you keep your job.

No progress, no challenge. No creativity. No way to express yourself.

That's what people are most happy with in life: when they have the work where they feel they can express themselves and have some creativity, and be involved. That they're challenged in a way that keeps the energy moving, rather than just come in, go home, come in, go home, gossip about people, talk about the TV shows, sports, etc.

Remember, how to practice... Our lives and the practice run parallel. A martial arts practice always parallels life.

How about quantity? What is quantity about again? As we covered in the chapter on the "Q's": quantity versus quality. What's different? Quantity tends to be superficial. Quantity is getting bored really quickly with anything that takes some work.

You know, the Jack-of-all-trades, master of none. This person never really gets deep with anything. Never really focuses on anything. Never becomes great at anything.

Never stands out.

"I just do it." Why? "I don't know, I just like it." There is very little substance there, and it can easily lose its luster.

Students get excited about learning new techniques in class. They light up. More show up when they hear they're going to learn something new. They love to be entertained. Otherwise, making an effort to get there is a little more difficult.

Those who think that way end up with nothing more than a superficial knowledge of anything.

Quality is depth. Quality is taking one thing and understanding every angle about that one thing. Quality is that path to mastery.

Quality is that mechanic everybody wants, who's got no time because he's so good, as opposed to the those who are starving for work, spending a fortune on advertising, because they do things half-heartedly. The positive side of pride is always doing your absolute best and being willing to stand by it.

How much time is wasted when you have to do a job or project more than once because you didn't give your full attention the first time?

Think about work and jobs. How can you progress in getting more raises and better positions and just moving up in your career without continuously improving and learning more?

Those who jump from job to job rarely get anywhere. They're lucky to even be able to pay their bills. Mastery can only come through consistent effort over time.

Relationships are the same. Jumping from person to person to person. What is a relationship to you? Is it joy? But only for you? Or is it about sharing and growing together? Is it to have a family and raise that family together, and grow in life together? Or is it just something convenient for you?

Would you prefer a quality relationship or a quantity of relationships, going from person to person without experiencing any real depth?

Quantity is the dabbler. Little this, little that. No depth.

Be Like The Bamboo

There's an old story of a bamboo shoot, a young bamboo shoot, who heard it's impossible to reach the sky. And this young bamboo shoot says, "Well, I'm going for it! I'm going to make it. I'm going to get farther than anyone ever got." And so, he's young, he's strong, and he believes he can do anything.

So he goes for it, and what he finds is the higher he grows, the more he bows.

Pride Loses, Humility Wins.

You know the competitor who wins and thinks he's so good he becomes complacent and no longer trains as seriously or tries as hard. The one who loses stays hungry, tries harder, keeps pushing, and thinking, "Got to get better!"

Think about that. If you never think you're good, you're always able to learn.

There's a story about a martial artist who climbed a mountain to meet a great master and asks, "I wonder if you have anything to teach me?" He then proceeds to tell him all he knows, "I've been to this master, and that master, and the other master... I trained very hard and learned a lot. I've spent five years at this famous dojo, three years with another great teacher, and I won this regional tournament and that national tournament." He then gets up to demonstrate and show off his skills, "I know this... and this... and I know how to..."

As he goes on showing off and bragging about all his experience and accomplishments, the master is serving him tea. He continues to talk, and the master continues pouring the tea. Then the tea starts overflowing out of the cup. He says, "Hey!

Don't you see what you're doing old man? Aren't you aware? You're overflowing the cup! Stop pouring!"

The master says, "This is just like your head. It's already full. I have nothing to teach you. Get out of here."

The Art of Change

Consider all the qualities discussed here. We talked about finding that special place for yourself. There was patience and perseverance. We talked about being fully present and that you've got to push yourself to make progress.

We've already discussed having passion with purpose and still maintaining a passive attitude, so you don't get too caught up in the results. Let them come when they come. Some things take time.

Just like when the kids ask, "Are we there yet? How much longer?" It takes how long it takes. Enjoy the ride.

I can't say that enough because as soon as something happens in your life that you don't like and you ask, "Why? Why? Why?" getting all upset and angry. But it doesn't help. It doesn't change anything. It only makes you feel worse.

Sure, it's normal for emotions to flow, but get past it and realize, "I can't control that." Instead ask yourself, "What *can* I do now?"

Life is a practice. Be it good or bad, no matter what happens, it's an experience. Every decision, no matter how large or how small, affects your path and what you're going to experience next. There are no small decisions. Each one affects what's going to happen next.

That's why, if you make decisions that help you go deeper into something, maybe you become better at the kind of work you do and get promoted. Or, to have a better relationship you learn more about how to have better relationships.

You can bring more quality to your life.

You make decisions that are going to help you understand your practice more. When you're out there training, are you focused? Are you fully present? The decisions in the moment; getting up, being lazy, not going to practice.

First thing in the morning, you might think, "I should go out and practice..." and then you turn over, and you don't bother.

And every time you decide, "I'm a little too tired to go to class today," every time you make that decision you take yourself further away from what you wanted when you got started.

Every time you don't take care of personal things, it starts interfering with your work. Now you're having problems at work. Procrastination and poor decisions are like cancer. It can spread into everything.

It's all these little things. Are they good or bad? I don't know. You don't know. It's all just an experience, but we are aligning so much of what we experience with all the little things we either do or don't do.

Are you making quality decisions or superficial, surface type decisions?

The point of a practice such as the discipline of Kung Fu is about recognizing who we are, where we came from, why we think the way we do, why we do what we do.

Then if we're happy with the results we're getting, keep going. If you're not so sure, you're not that happy, you're not at peace, maybe not so healthy, etc. The realization allows you to make adjustments to your course. You must think, say, and do things differently if you want to experience anything different.

What's the definition of insanity? Doing the same thing over and over and expecting different results.

Life is a practice. We can make adjustments. We are not stuck, we just think we are. We think sometimes we make a decision and that's the end. Not so. Small steps in the right direction add up to better results.

Recognize what you need to learn or why you do what you do, and what you can change about that. It's not going to happen overnight, but it will happen.

Either way, you're changing, whether you like it or not. You're getting older. Are you getting wiser? Most people are just in a pattern, sleepwalking through life. If you wake up and realize you want something different, and you're not too proud to change, you can. Even if you just start with little changes in the right direction (meaning "right" for what you want).

Maybe you need to have courage and get a new job, even in a bad economy. You might think, "I can't because of this economy..." But maybe that's exactly what you need! Maybe you'd be happier. Maybe you'd be more satisfied in a different kind of work environment. Maybe you would do better in a whole different field.

There are people who studied for years on their own to learn another field. It might not take years. If you're really interested in something, you can get there.

You can get there with consistent effort over time.

Want your relationships to be better? Remember why you got together in the first place. Remember what that relationship really means to you. What was exciting about this person? Have you stifled the very person you love? Because you want them to fit into what you think the world should be?

Many forget how and why they fell in love in the first place. Being more aware of what we do allows us to adjust ourselves and to begin supporting those we love to be who they are and express themselves as they choose so they too can be creative and enjoy their lives.

Because if your partner in life is happy, aren't you going to be happier, too? I'm sure you've heard the saying, "Happy wife, happy life."

We have so much more control of our inner world and therefore can affect our outer world, but we have to realize what we do and why we do it first. That's why the highest level goal in the martial arts is to *discover the ego... then destroy it.*

Pride makes this impossible with the limiting beliefs of who you think you are. Pride stagnates growth.

Humility makes anything possible, with never-ending possibilities.

I don't know what I don't know. And I always reserve the right to change my mind if my experience reveals a conflict with what I previously thought to be true.

PART FOUR

A Lifetime of Return on Investment

In the financial world, learning just the right thing to do with your money and investments can provide a lifetime of ROI. Get the right tip from the right person at the right time, and for a lifetime of return on your investment, you'd put in everything to take advantage of the opportunity.

I find the same benefit in the martial arts. The more you invest in training your body and mind, the more you will enjoy the benefits for a lifetime.

It truly is the gift that keeps on giving and an experience that changes the lives of those who are willing to put in the time and effort.

Seriously, how much would it be worth it to you if you knew at the other end you'd be happier and healthier while feeling stronger, more settled, less emotional, and more confident?

Imagine a practice, a discipline, that leads to better relationships, more job security and career advancement, an easier time learning and a habit of following through on your pursuits. One that also helps to keep you and those you care about safer simply because of a whole new mindset and approach to your life that is a consequence of proper practice.

All because you've exposed yourself to a new way of thinking, of moving, and of living.

What would you be willing to invest? What would you be willing to sacrifice if you knew you could not fail as long as you just keep going?

Those in our past have given up more than you could imagine in many cases. Many risked prison or even death to learn what they knew was a way to personal empowerment and a better life.

CHAPTER 24

Be Willing To Do This
To Reach Your Full Potential

Modern living is so full of conveniences that it can be hard to imagine going out of your way to learn something.

If you're serious about any activity, be it baseball, basketball, tennis, art or music, why not do everything in your power to train with the best?

The best are the best for a reason. They know things that the average person does not. They know what it takes to be great at what they do.

They know how you can get there too.

How Far Are You Willing To Go For What You Want To Learn?

My Grand-Shifu, Lu Shui Tian, sought out the best Ba Gua Zhang master he could find, which turned out to be two days away on horseback! *Two days on horseback to get to his teacher*. And there was no Holiday Inn for the overnight.

Today in the martial arts industry, where school owners learn how to have a successful martial arts business, they say you really only have about a three to five-mile radius.

Lu Shui Tian rode two days on horseback, camping out on the side of the road during the trip, to get to his teacher. When people really want to learn, how important is it? What are they willing to go through? What are they willing to do?

They do whatever it takes.

If you really want to learn something, anything, you have this choice. You can do whatever it takes. Don't cut yourself short and always settle for what's convenient.

If you really, really want it, you can have it. You just have to be willing.

Are you worth it?

Getting Started With A Traditional Teacher

When my Shifu, Bok-Nam Park, was young he was a bit of a trouble-maker. He had a tendancy to run with the wrong crowd. So at one point his father gave him a choice – martial arts or college. The young Park wanted martial arts.

So his father found a famous Chinese martial arts master who was right there in the Chinatown section of Incheon, the same city where the Park family lived. This master was none other than Lu Shui Tian, who was very well known in the Chinese community. They knew if you want to learn Kung Fu, he was the one to see.

So the young Park goes and knocks on the master's door, and says, "I would like to learn martial arts with you. I'd like to practice with you," and Lu Shui Tian closes the door in his face.

What would you do next if you really wanted to learn from this person?

The next day the young Park returns. He knocks on the door again. "Please, I want to learn martial arts with you!" and the master again closes the door on his face.

Apparently, this went on every day for a month!

You see, his mind was made up. "I want to practice. My father gave me this choice. I want to prove I can do this."

So he returns and does the same thing every day until he finally starts to become discouraged the last couple of days. He begins to think, "Maybe he just doesn't want to teach me because I'm Korean." All his students were Chinese. Not an impossible scenario. He said to himself, "Maybe I should give up."

It was then that he was finally invited in - as if the master knew.

Have you had similar experiences in your own life? You meet the right person at the right time who leads you to your career or your spouse or an investment that pays off and leads to a life decision that you may never have been able to make otherwise. Or that phone call out of the blue, just when you were thinking of that person or something you needed from the caller.

Life is funny that way.

"Come on in. You can come here." Of course, he wasn't speaking English, but he says, "Come in. You can come to the class." There were only about 10 or 15 students.

The master says, "You can come here. Sit down." It seems like he was being nice now, but he wasn't nice at all. And that was that. So everybody's practicing, and the young Park is just sitting there watching. Everybody finishes, and the master says "Clean up!" That was about it. That also went on for about a month.

Everybody's practicing, he just sits there, watches, and cleans up afterward. In fact, my teacher says that one time when a storm was coming, and he wanted to quickly clean up, the Great-Grandmaster Lu says, "Sit!" He made him sit and wait until the storm was really bad. Then he said, "Now, clean up!" right in the middle of the storm.

He wasn't a very nice guy.

The Old Way, *Always Testing*

You see, the traditional teacher was testing. Which was why my teacher knew even back then, "Oh, this is a very traditional teacher. Every day he's just testing me." People knew this was the norm. And if you really wanted to practice with someone like that it was the student's job to prove they were worthy.

In China and other East Asian countries where these traditional martial arts originated, and in education in general, it was always the student's responsibility to learn.

In the West, we tend to put the burden on the teacher. If the students aren't getting it the teacher is blamed and maybe even fired in academia.

The answer lies somewhere in-between. The teacher should do everything in his or her power to provide the best learning experience for the student so that unnecessary time isn't wasted (and each generation isn't trying to reinvent the wheel!). The arts can never progress like that and truth be told, these arts are unfortunately *regressing*.

Is it because of the teachers or the students? I'd say it's a bit of both. I recognize that it is impossible to "get it" without personal experience through "eating bitter" and one's own "dirt time." However, I am always looking for ways to help my students make real progress in less time with more efficient practice. That's the reality of modern day living. Because people are generally overwhelmed with so much to keep up with time is now at more of a premium than at any other time in history.

Today's challenges are just as intense in their own way as those of the past. Different times bring different challenges to learning something of great value that can result in your life never being the same.

People only have so much time these days, and these traditional arts are far too valuable for me not to give it every effort to make sure the next generation (and generations to come) also can obtain the full benefits.

I owe that to future generations because of what those who came before me have gone through and done for me and my life.

It's the very reason why I've written this book. It's for you to get a glimpse of the possibilities in store for you.

You Have A Problem? There's the Door.

My teacher's father wanted his son to learn discipline because he knew he was the type to get in trouble. He knew his son got into a lot of fights, and he wanted to straighten him out. It was common in Asia that young people were brought to the martial artist, to those Shifu's or Sensei's, to learn how to live in this world, not just for fighting. Park already could fight. For years he had been boxing and was a black belt in Tang Soo Do.

Did he learn to fight even better with Ba Gua? Yeah, much better, he says, but that wasn't the reason his father wanted him to train with the Chinese master.

He wanted his son to learn discipline. And of course, when he told Lu Shui Tian, well, Lu took it to the extreme, including the strategic use of a cane.

Anytime he did something wrong, the young Park got hit with the cane. This is the old traditional training, and the master would always watch the young Park's face to see his reaction. They might be sitting there having tea, and he would just get up and whack him. Then he would observe the response.

Does he get angry? Does he cry? How much self-control does he have? There was constant testing.

That Was Then This Is Now

Today you would never allow someone to treat you like that! If you were enrolled in a martial arts school and the teacher hit you with a cane he'd probably be brought up on charges!

And you'd go down the street or be done with martial arts altogether due to the bad experience.

But that's how important it was for people like my teacher. They put up with whatever they had to in order to learn what they wanted.

The point here is that although it is unlikely that a teacher will do such things to their students today, a good teacher does not make it easy at all.

If the students' experience and the actual progress that manifests in their day-to-day lives are important to the teacher, then he or she must create a new modern day environment that brings the same or similar results.

The training must challenge the student mentally, emotionally, and spiritually, as well as physically. Advancement should never be automatic or on any artificially created timetable.

That is cheating the student.

Would you want to receive a rank that may actually mean nothing at all? Only when you are truly challenged and overcome that challenge, do you grow.

Here's a favorite poem of mine:

Good Timber

by Douglas Malloch

The tree that never had to fight
For sun and sky and air and light,
But stood out in the open plain
And always got its share of rain,
Never became a forest king
But lived and died a scrubby thing.

The man who never had to toil
To gain and farm his patch of soil,
Who never had to win his share
Of sun and sky and light and air,
Never became a manly man
But lived and died as he began.

Good timber does not grow with ease:
The stronger wind, the stronger trees;
The further sky, the greater length;
The more the storm, the more the strength.
By sun and cold, by rain and snow,
In trees and men good timbers grow.

Where thickest lies the forest growth,
We find the patriarchs of both.
And they hold counsel with the stars
Whose broken branches show the scars
Of many winds and much of strife.
This is the common law of life.

We Appreciate More When We Have Less

When I trained with Dr. Yang Jwing-Ming back in the 80's and early 90's, he would tell me about his students in Poland and how they were "so much better than the American students" because *they appreciated practicing.*

They didn't have anything else. They didn't have all the distractions we have. They didn't live this busy, busy, busy life like we do here in the U.S. Dr. Yang would travel and teach there, and all they wanted was to be able to learn and practice. So he would come back to the United States, and just kind of shake his head and tell the story about how "they're very serious over there."

People have a hard time today appreciating and realizing what the people who have earned and enjoyed the greatest returns were willing to go through to get there. It's difficult to relate to what they were willing to sacrifice to learn real martial arts.

Grandmaster Park came to Lu Shui Tian at 17-years-old. He wasn't allowed to have a girlfriend for five years. No dating at all. He could only see his friends on Sunday. That was it. Can you imagine?

"You want to do this or not?" That was his choice. Lights on, lights off. There was no in-between. No, "come when you feel like it." This is what we're doing. You practice. That's it. No girlfriend, no distractions. That was it.

It's very easy at that age to get distracted. You go off, get in trouble, or whatever... "No! I don't want to waste my time," he would think, and say to himself, "You do this right, or you don't do it at all."

Today, it's very different. Every town usually has a couple of martial arts schools. Go online, do a search. You get all kinds of schools. There are many different styles and choices. And now, because of an industry that is mastering marketing in business, people are being sold a bill of goods based on emotions. Rather than the quality they offer, they just know how to present it, so you think it's great.

"You can be a black belt!"

But what will it be worth?

You have no way of judging the quality anymore. Not if you don't know what to look for. And if it isn't extremely convenient... "Uh, no thanks."

Remember the three to five-mile radius. In our dojang we have more adults in an industry dominated by children. We also have people from further than that "industry standard," and I've had people coming from up to two hours away regularly and now even from outside of the country who come and spend time when they can, like the old days, because they see something different than what they find locally or what's convenient.

It would be nice if more martial arts schools would take these things into consideration. People want the real experience more than being sold on a black belt. Then more would benefit from what these arts have to offer.

When I was with Dr. Yang Jwing-Ming, he was in Boston. I was in northern New Jersey. I used to go there monthly, leaving about 4AM to make the early class and stay overnight, on the floor in the school, so I could train privately with Dr. Yang early Sunday morning.

With Shifu Park, it was a three-and-a-half-hour drive to Baltimore, fifty times a year, every Saturday. That was my Saturday. That was it. Fifty times a year. And then Richmond, a couple of times a year, where he had his "headquarters." I'd follow wherever he went to teach, because I really wanted to learn.

There was no social life, but I must say, it has been well worth it. I wouldn't trade it for anything.

In the old times, students would choose and make the effort based on the teacher, not the convenience. Even a two-day ride on horseback, each way, and sleeping on the side of the road, was worth it.

There's so much more than just punching and kicking. You can learn that anywhere.

Today, if there is even a little inconvenience here come the excuses. "They're too hard." "They're too far." "They're too expensive."

I've trained with some of the most difficult teachers in the most difficult Chinese martial art style (Ba Gua Zhang is known in China as "graduate school"). I have traveled all over the country and even outside the country. I couldn't possibly figure out how much it has cost me financially, (well over $100,000 I'm sure), but the truth is it didn't *cost* me anything because it was an investment in myself and my life. By far, it has been the best investment I have ever made.

All because I never let location, expense or difficulty learning get in the way of what I wanted.

You can too if you so choose. Then you will have something that makes your life so much more powerful.

These arts have been changing lives since ancient times.

CHAPTER 25

"But I Just Want To Be Healthy..."

Should those who are most interested in health and taking classes for meditation and Qigong care about any of this? Should it matter what others have gone through?

In some ways, it reminds me of when I was a child and didn't want to eat my vegetables or finish my plate, my mother would say, "Finish your food! Don't you know there are children starving in Africa?!?"

Yes, Mom, I know, because you tell me every night.

Did it get me to eat my food? Rarely. I'd just say, "Can I give it to them?"

So why does any of this matter? What's the difference?

There was a time when these arts were a closely guarded secret. In fact, many teachers still protect the deeper meanings, only reluctantly providing the seeds of growth that won't sprout without proper care (diligent practice).

That's how it was learning from my Shifu.

They had to give up so much if they wanted to learn. They had to work through years of blood, sweat, and tears in order to truly comprehend it. They developed a strong appreciation for the journey.

They don't want these arts to become handicapped by half-hearted efforts that result in little understanding or benefit to the practitioner.

So, if you really want to learn then developing the same appreciation for where it came from, enhances your ability to reap the reward of what you sow.

You'll simply try harder.

One thing I always took to heart is respecting the time and effort that my teacher was putting into teaching me. I would do everything in my power to not have to be told the same thing twice.

On the nearly four-hour drive home I would review what we did in my mind.

When I arrived home, I would journal what we did, which would help me to go through the class again in my mind.

If there were some new physical movements, I would walk through them again physically before going to bed.

And I would physically go through it again in the morning.

I would not wait until I had the perfect time to have a full practice. By the time I did, it would be clear, and I'd be able to practice it right.

It has been my experience that not only does this save time in the long run, because my understanding of what I am doing increases faster, the benefits also grow exponentially.

Practicing right is not just physical. It is also a mindset. Practice right and your health and fitness levels will go through the roof.

Facing Adversity

It is the depth of the detail that these arts contain and the tendency to regularly face adversity that makes traditional martial arts special.

Adversity is naturally built into the learning process as it becomes "you against you" many times in frustration.

Growing beyond what is comfortable is not easy.

And then there is partner work, where there are so many different kinds of people to learn to work with (not against).

Just like in your everyday life, traditional martial arts have a way of always challenging you.

It's not just about punching and kicking to music like the old "Tae Bo" or "cardio kickboxing" exercise.

Many have been sold on kickboxing to music and actually think they can defend themselves with it. Because they're punching and kicking a free-standing "heavy bag," getting their workout in, they think they can defend themselves. How many people have been sold on that?

If you've chosen martial arts to get in shape because you want to actually learn something useful while you get in your exercise, then why not do the real thing?

What makes real martial arts so powerful is the fact that in order to develop real skills it takes full engagement with consistent effort over time. You really have to focus. Without the details, you don't know what to focus on. There is no other way, and there are no shortcuts.

And so, you lose the most profound effects of the practice, the very thing that changes lives by powerfully impacting everything from your work, to your relationships, to your health, to your ability to learn and grow in life.

Because the real thing trains your body *and your mind.*

I can't stress that enough.

Empty Without Meaning

The forms, which can be anything from a single technique to an elaborate sequence of techniques, are empty without the essence of the training, without the training of all the components, without the development of the mind, the breath, and the body fully, those forms are useless. It becomes just a dance when practiced like that. It's very sad that people think otherwise because they are really missing out (and rarely even know it!).

There are many who think that the traditional forms are a useless waste of time.

For over 40 years in China these arts were taught without the fighting applications due to communist law against practicing anything related to fighting.

Many have learned and then passed these sequences down without the deeper and more complete knowledge of what is contained within. Adding fancy components so it looks good in demonstrations and tournaments also began to take precendance over multiple generations. The forms are useless for self defense like that because they're empty. The true meaning is lost.

But the real traditional forms, done right and with all the components developed over years, become a collection of what has been shown to work through experience. These traditional sequences are very much like an encyclopedia holding all the information you need and a way to pass it down, intact, from generation to generation.

How do you know a good martial art? Is it how beautiful or fancy it is? No, not at all. In fact, traditional forms may not be pretty at all for demonstration. Most of the practice is internal (mindset, breath, and movement coordination).

How about one or two forms that eventually include everything you need? (By "eventually" I mean that as your understanding increases more meaning is discovered and more benefit is realized. Same form, different you.)

What can you possibly do with a hundred or two hundred, or three hundred different forms? It's a waste of time that actually makes it more difficult to ever become highly skilled. Your whole focus becomes remembering rather than the profound experience.

Once again, that's the "Jack of all trades, master of none."

The reason why many teachers need so many forms is because it's the only way they know how to keep people interested. It probably was the only way they kept themselves interested!

Always focusing on "What's next?" rather than "What's now?" is an endless road to nowhere.

Training Our Youth

I'll teach a good number more *Shaolin Long Fist Kung Fu* sequences to the children and teens in our dojang than I teach adults because it fulfills the desire for more variety and having the sense of learning something new.

It's a wonderful art that keeps them interested because of all the exciting things they get exposed to from empty hand to weapons to flying kicks and joint locks. There is no shortage of information to absorb!

Long Fist is also an excellent foundation for learning any other Kung Fu style because the student gets exposed to numerous variations of body movements and traditional techniques that gradually require more and more coordination.

It is an increasingly challenging physical art. Young people have a lot of fun while learning a whole gamut of skills and developing a strong, supple and coordinated body with a focused mind.

In addition to being able to learn a lot of variety, so much of it is the same things done different ways. The style is excellent for kids and teens because it naturally disguises repetition so they can become well-skilled without becoming bored.

Since it is my perspective that everything we practice should be like a form of meditation, the kids also practice sitting meditation, now proven in numerous studies to be of great benefit for kids (bit.ly/forbes-meditation-benefits-children).

Meditation is even being used in detention these days! (bit.ly/cnn-meditation-in-schools)

As the phrase we adopted from my good friend and amazing teacher Sifu* Robert Brown in the Detroit, MI area expresses so well: "Meditation is the foundation of all true martial arts." Every martial arts school should seriously consider this.

Making Rank

I'm not very interested in passing people along just so they're happy. That would be cheating them of discovering what they're capable of. And no one knows what they're capable of until they're truly challenged.

For the ones who do the work and stick it out, it shows. They're phenomenal. It's a beautiful thing to witness what I see in the youth program from the ones who are willing to stick it out and do the work.

A Never Ending Pursuit Full of Personal Discovery

Whatever it is we're teaching, whatever it is we're doing, whatever level you're at, you have things that you have to tweak and focus on and practice more.

When something hurts, it's because generally there's a weakness there or there's something you're doing in your normal day-to-day activities (or lack of activities) that's causing a problem. *So work on that more.* For those who really want to acquire these skills, that's the only way.

For example, one thing I discovered from experience: The more you sit, the more you need to squat or practice the stance known as *Pu Bu,* the "squat stance" (squatting with one leg extended to the side - a bit like a side lunge, but all the way down with both feet flat) because those are the joints (and muscles, tendons, ligaments, etc.) that get the stiffest.

Knowing and applying things like that in your life can make a big difference in what you experience as you age.

We *can* age gracefully and maintain optimal health.

Now that's a lifetime of return on investment!

CHAPTER 26

———◆———

Without This, It is Virtually Impossible to Improve Your Life

Don't just mindlessly go through the various exercises. As you become more advanced, this is practice by prescription.

If you know what you need, you can practice by prescription. In life, utilize your strengths but work on your weaknesses. That is the path to mastery.

Also, knowing *why* you personally practice gives direction, as discussed in Part Three. What is most important for you to get out of it?

I've always thought the fighting side would be to become so skilled that you never have to fight and if you had no choice you could get control of that fight, possibly without hurting someone.

Of course, no one can guarantee that. Until you're in that moment, you have no idea what you have to do. But you may be able to choose to hurt them in a way that disables them as opposed to killing or permanently maiming them.

The skilled person with the focused and calm mind can make those choices under duress. That's one far end of the spectrum.

At the other end of the spectrum in traditional martial arts practice is sitting on a cushion or a chair in meditation.

Your life is everywhere in-between. All the things you face all the time.

How often do you face a guy in the back alley with a knife? Did you have a fight today, yesterday, a month ago, or a year ago? Ever? Most people completely misunderstand the purpose of training the fighting side of the art.

In addition to the obvious (self defense), the real purpose is *to discover who you are* and *to master yourself.*

How Do You Respond?

When you spar, when you put yourself in harm's way physically, you learn how to respond to adversity, to challenges, real challenges. Then you can up the ante depending on your level and how much you've practiced. As your skills improve, you can take on bigger challenges.

Because you're not the same person you were before.

If you get hit, how do you respond?

Do you freak out, get angry, cry, or feel the need to get them back?

Or can you just take responsibility, re-evaluate and be grateful you now know what to work on?

This experience is unique to martial arts and can be *very revealing* as it exposes the truth about you.

Can you handle the truth? Without it, it is virtually impossible to improve your life.

How you respond to challenges in the dojang is exactly how you respond to any adversity in your life.

Do you tend to overreact when things don't go your way? No matter how justified you think you are, does it really help or make things worse?

Remember, the only thing we can definitely control is ourselves. But in order to work on this, we have to know where we're starting from.

If you're at a mall looking at the directory and trying to find a particular store you want to go to, what's the first thing you have to find?

You have to find that little sticker that says, "You are here."

Without a reference for where you're starting from, you'll have no way to get where you want to go.

Controlled By Emotions

The average person is controlled by their emotions. We want to have control of our emotions. Having a better understanding of our shortcomings and appreciation for our challenges allows us to learn and grow.

When we practice, when my teacher practiced, when those students in Poland practice, all the examples I gave, that month of knocking on the door, the willingness to sit and watch and not be able to take part, how strong was their will to learn? Why? Because they knew if they acquired the skills that the master had their life would be better because of it.

Can you appreciate that? Personally, I am eternally grateful that my teacher went through the trials and tribulations that he did so that I, in turn, could learn them too. In fact, I am inspired by it.

Sure, it's no fun when you're going through it, and most will think to change roads before they ever really get anywhere, but that's why so few are actually great at anything. Greatness is a habit.

And how you do anything is how you do everything.

The real question is: what are you willing to go through to learn and become more than you are now?

And if you mastered yourself, your body, your breath, your mind and your emotions, what would your life be like?

For me it's a privilege to have the opportunity to learn these tools and techniques which have been proven over many generations to change lives for the better. Therefore, it's my responsibility to practice them so I can fully experience their effects.

To dedicate myself to this practice is to show appreciation for what I have learned and for those who took the time to share this art with me. There are not many things I know of that can have such a positive impact on the life of a serious student.

Those who do what it takes change physically, mentally, emotionally, and spiritually. And please don't get caught up on "spiritually" because anything you make special, anything you focus on, anything you put your all into, *you make sacred.* You make it spiritual.

There is nothing we can do in this world that isn't spiritual. It's just a matter of how focused we are on what we're doing and how connected we are to it.

Whatever you fully engage yourself in, you'll get good at. As you get good, you get the benefits. You get those things you want, the little things, you know, the things like "I want more confidence." "I want to lose weight." "I want to be in better shape." All those things and so much more.

Words only go so far because everybody has their own story. During our testing process for a student, we get to see a little bit about that story. A lot of people end up in tears, and there is an opportunity to release the sort of things that may have been bottled up inside. It's a very real experience. You can't fake that.

It's so real it touches the soul. It changes people. Then as you're changed, and you're not the same anymore, you don't act the same. You've become someone new. People will notice, and they might ask about it.

That's why the greatest gift you can give to the art, the way to demonstrate that you understand the privilege of learning it, is to practice to a point where you really are a martial artist in everything you do. Then you become a positive influence in your life, and other people want to practice because of what they see in you.

What better gift can you give to the world than to be a positive and inspiring influence? You can be the example because the practice works. You just have to do the work consistently, over time.

I recently heard a quote from Walt Disney:

"Do what you do so well that other people, when they see you, when they see it, they want to come and see it again. And they want to bring their friends to see, too."

You see, that is the essence of a martial artist, "Do what you do so well..." I don't care if you're an accountant, you're an engineer, you're a salesperson, you drive a taxi, whatever you do, you do it so well that others notice and talk about it.

Detail Oriented

I just had a major problem with my motorcycle and brought it to the dealer to work on it. I was pleasantly surprised by the level of detail the mechanic displayed.

I ride in all kinds of weather and most who ride don't. Most just ride on beautiful days but when you ride in the rain dirt gets kicked up on wet roads and gets in everything.

He went and cleaned it all out. He figured everything out to such a degree that I will always ask for him again. This guy is my mechanic, without question. I want him working on that thing because other people might have me stuck 3,000 miles away one day. Not a nice ride.

Can you be like that in what you do? You should never have a shortage of work when people know you care that much.

That's the martial artist - applying it to everything you do, as a parent, as an employer, employee, whatever. Be the best 'you' you can be, and the practice is the ultimate act of *sharpening the saw*.

Sharpening Your Saw

Imagine a competition between two lumberjacks. They each stand at opposite sides of the road they need to cut down. One lumberjack is big and strong, and he can work through the day and night just going and going. He's so strong, and he can keep it up.

The second lumberjack only works about a third of the time and nobody can figure out how he's still ahead of the big, strong lumberjack who's working day and night.

At the end of the competition they ask him, "How did you win so easily working only one-third of the time of your competition?" He says, "Well, the other two-thirds of the time, I was sharpening my saw."

You see, martial arts is just like that: self-perfection. Never get there, keep working on it. You see some issue with a relationship, you need to fix it in yourself. How can I be a little better this way or that?

He or she is always working on it by practicing physically, sitting and meditating, getting fully engaged in everything they do, completely and utterly focused.

With regular practice, these things become part of you. You can't help but apply them to everything you do.

Change the World

Do you want to change the world or do you just complain about the world? Complaining doesn't help. If you want to change the world, realize how many people you touch on a regular basis.

If you practice and become that better person, that better you, more centered and calmer, you'll be more open to helping other people excel and rooting for their success rather than becoming jealous, the ugliest emotion.

You'll want people to do well. You'll feel good for them when you are truly confident, regardless of your circumstances. Real confidence comes from real practice. It comes from real training.

That's how you change the world. People who see you, they see you're happy, they see you're peaceful, and then they want to be more like you.

The words of Gandhi are appropriate here, "Be the change you wish to see in the world."

Pay It Forward

What's the best gift you can give in appreciation to the great martial artists of the past who did what they needed to do then handed down these incredible tools to improve the human condition? Do what you need to do as they did. Then pay it forward by your influence and ability to make the world a better place.

Remember, it takes how long it takes. Just like it takes a different number of years for each of us to be fully grown, we do not each progress the same way in the same amount of time.

Again, in my experience, it's well worth it. Life can be long or short. We really don't know. I'd rather be well-prepared for a long one (so it's a great one) by investing daily, just in case.

In 2016, I hit the age of fifty, with thirty-three years of continuous practice as of this writing.

To this day, I continue to train and research. Wherever I need to travel, whatever I need to do or how cold or hot it is where we're training, I will do it in order to keep evolving myself, so I can bring my students as much as I can of what these arts have to offer.

I sincerely want the very best for my students, and I don't know what I don't know. There's no resting on laurels for me.

I haven't slowed one bit as my passion for this practice and what it can do for people is at least as strong as ever. Maybe stronger as I am continually inspired by what I see in the many students in our dojang who show up regularly and continue to do the work. As their lives change for the better and I see the joy in their expression as they "get it," there really is no better reward.

I have such reverence for those who came before me and respect for these arts that I want nothing more than to be able to give the very best to my students so that they, in turn, can one day pass it on to the next generation and beyond. This can only happen by their first-hand experience and their own deep understanding.

My pledge is to continue to do all I can to make that a reality.

* Is it *Shifu* or *Sifu*? This is the same title, either way it is spelled. Some choose the Cantonese spelling, some choose the Mandarin, and *Pinyin*, spelling. I chose the Mandarin version years ago, and prefer Pinyin whenever writing Chinese words as it is now the standard in China. The Chinese characters are the same. According to Wikipedia, "It is used as a title for and role of a skillful person or master."

See more about what this term means to me in the next chapter...

PART FIVE

A New Perspective

People whose perspective of martial arts training as all about fighting in order for it to be practical simply don't understand the profound depth of these arts.

It's far easier to buy a gun and learn how to shoot so you can protect yourself. If you just want to be able to hurt someone, there are far easier ways. Why spend so much time, energy and expense on learning such a difficult art?

To me, the most practical training not only teaches you how to physically defend yourself but also how to avoid the fight altogether. We need a very different perspective in order to do this successfully, and that is what this section is about.

The section is about how we each view and respond to the world around us.

It will change some beliefs about things like respect, freedom, and why you experience the world the way you do.

The story about The Blind Men and the Elephant displays how we think we're right but only see things from where we stand.

There's a bit about fear, optimism vs. pessimism, and your attitude toward things.

We end this section with a few words about The Power Inside you.

CHAPTER 27

———◆———

We Don't See Things As They Are

We don't see things as they are. We see things as we think
they are.

Give that some thought.

You only can see from your perspective. It's the way you see
things and how you approach them. It has a strong correlation
with your attitude.

At the Blue Dragon School of Martial Arts, where I teach
the traditional Chinese martial art, Ba Gua Zhang, our training
is never just about practicing physical martial arts (punching,
kicking, grappling, etc.). Everything must transfer into our
lives, or it's not very useful.

These arts, when taught and practiced properly, are
disciplines that have a profound positive and empowering
impact on all those who do the work. This is the real Kung Fu.

Change Your Thinking

How can any of us improve or change if we get too caught up in being good enough or right about something?

I've been blessed with an attitude that tells me I'm never good enough. Psychologists might say that is not the healthy way to think of yourself as they tell their clients, "You ARE good enough!"

The difference is I always believe that I can be better and do better. I'm less concerned with being right and more concerned with improving my life and the lives of others. If I see a better way, I will take it, and give it all I've got.

I've been wrong many times before. The thing is I don't identify myself with what I believe. If I'm wrong and discover a better way, I'll change and let anyone who follows me know that I've changed, and why. The last thing I'd want to do is keep trying to make the wrong way right to "save face" as they say in the East.

A Different Perspective of Respect

Possibly the most powerful lesson I've learned through all my years of martial arts and taking more of a Daoist approach to life is about respect.

It's been said that the martial arts begin and end with respect.

Usually, when I hear people talk about respect, it's about the other person deserving respect. It's about showing the other that you respect them so that they feel respected.

Many will go out of their way trying to accomplish things so that they get respect. And they're very disappointed if not angry if they don't think they are getting the respect they deserve.

They might ask with anger, "What do I have to do?!?" and live their whole life pursuing this evasive feeling of being respected.

For many, it's like a reward or even a requirement. Respect your seniors. Respect your elders. Respect your superiors. Respect your teachers. Respect authority.

And if you don't, it can cause you an awful lot of trouble.

That's great. No argument is being offered here. It's just that I see it and approach it a whole different way. In fact, I flip it on its head.

Let Me Explain, From the Seat of a Harley...

Most of the miles I travel are on a motorcycle. Many times on the highway, I've had a car come right into my lane. They clearly did not see me.

What's more important for me to hit at this point, the horn or the brake? (Or would you prefer a third option: the person driving the car that cut me off?)

My observation of the horn, especially having lived my whole life just outside of Manhattan/NYC, is that it's there to yell at people when you want them to move along or get out of your way, such as when the people behind you at a red light see that the crossroad traffic light has turned yellow. They want your engine roaring so you can get moving at full speed as the red turns to green. I can feel them saying, "C'mon already!!"

Rarely do I see it used as a warning, or what it was actually meant for. Unless they mean, "I'm warning you, get moving, or I'm going to get out of my car, come over there and kick your ass!"

In a real-life situation on the road, you don't have time to hit your horn. All you should be doing is hitting the brake, essentially defending yourself and responding in a way that keeps you safe. Your reflex should be the brake, not the horn.

Afterward, you can use your horn if you feel the need to yell at them!

That was a joke, of course. But isn't that exactly what we do?

It is where I come from.

Truth be told, I usually can't even find my horn because I never use it!

So let's get back to the point here: if someone cuts me off on the road because they didn't see me or know I was there, did they disrespect me?

No, they're just self-absorbed, distracted or simply not paying attention.

Have you ever cut off a biker? Have you ever cut off anyone? What happens next?

Many times they probably sped up to pass you with their horn honking and the bird in your face. They may even cut you off too! (Which is brilliant, really). But they have to get you back, right? They have to even the score.

Isn't it basically the same when a person doesn't hold the door for you, and it hits you in the face? Sure, it would be nice if they held it, but I doubt they did it on purpose. Don't get angry. Instead just make sure you don't let that door hit you in the face!

Again, they're just not paying attention. If I get hit with that door, I see it as my fault for also not paying attention. I don't believe yelling at them will fix anything. It will, however, make me more diligently aware going forward.

So I say, "Thank you," for the extra training, with a smile on my face.

And It's Not A Race!

Why are so many bothered, if not challenged, when someone passes them on the road? Why do people tend to speed up when someone puts on their blinker to change lanes?

I'm not saying I'm never guilty of it too, but it really is a strange phenomenon. Is this a demand for respect? Like saying, "I was first! I was in front of you! Stay back!"

Who cares really? Just do your best to get where you're going safely and in one piece. Worrying so much about what others are doing around you is just causing you more distress.

This is a very unwise and unproductive way to live. It certainly doesn't make anything better.

To me, respect is about what is in your mind. What is in your heart? What are your thoughts about the person? It's more about seeing the other person, the elder, the superior, the teacher as someone who is further down the road (the meaning of the Japanese title, "Sensei"), or someone who has worked really hard for their position having earned their knowledge and expertise.

Maybe they've just lived longer and know some things you don't simply because of time and experience. Maybe they're a little wiser.

Maybe they're not.

You see no one is better or worse than you, but just as special. They are just as unique, and they simply have another perspective to offer.

You can see them as another being having the experience of this world, another spark of the Divine, like yourself, who has all sorts of personal opinions and beliefs and experiences and are ultimately doing the best they know how to do. You can even have a sense of reverence for them.

Now, how does that feel?

The big question here is: do you respect them less if they don't respect you? If they don't show you respect, do you get upset or angry?

Someone cuts you off on the road. You're honking your horn. You're yelling at them. Your knuckles are white as you grip the steering wheel. Now you're upset. Now you're angry, emotional, and stressed.

Is that helping or making anything better? No, it's making you sick.

What's More Important, the Inner World or the Outer World?

What affects you more, inner or outer? Do your ways, your feelings, your emotions, your thoughts, your actions come from inside you or outside you, influenced by everything around you?

There is a saying that, "Environment is stronger than will." However, as a martial artist training myself every day, I would prefer to become stronger than the environment.

As I see it, a martial artist is not so influenced by those things around him that he knows he cannot control. He should be able to defend and protect himself and his loved ones and know how to keep them safe from harm if ever necessary.

He should know how to recognize when he has to defend and not have knee-jerk emotional reactions to protect his pride.

If someone is angry at me, I don't have to be angry back. I like the yin-yang concept: to be like water to the angry person's fire.

Don't worry about who's right.

If you respect others regardless of their actions or how they treat you and can still respect them as a human being, this is good for you as well as those around you. Now you're influencing the world around you in a more positive way.

And you're not so influenced by the negativity around you. No more blaming and complaining.

By developing yourself and becoming more confident, by believing in yourself, to the point that you are in control of your emotions, your thoughts and then your actions, you strengthen the inside and become less of a slave to what's happening around you.

What You Think and Say and Do Becomes You.

This includes what you say to others as well as what you say to yourself. Do you automatically show respect, or are you completely influenced by how the other acts first?

You can always be the one who shows respect. You can always be the one who is nice, especially when you have the confidence and root or grounding or know who you are. This is what results from proper training in traditional martial arts. It must include meditation, an integral component of traditional martial arts.

It's easy to imagine the old master sitting in meditation. So what happened with his students and grand-students?

Only with a calm and centered mind can you be in control of you.

That's why I said respect from the perspective described here is probably the most powerful thing I've learned through this practice.

If you get stressed because of what's going on around you on a day-to-day basis, due to the high demands of modern life hitting from so many directions at once, you will always be stressed. And most people are.

What could possibly end the stress? The world changing? The people in your life changing? People being nicer to you and changing their attitudes?

Good luck with that.

How much struggle, how much wasted energy and effort have you spent trying to change those around you?

That's why yelling at someone on the road because they didn't see you doesn't make any sense. You're upset. You may have upset them as well and now what? Did you change anything?

You can't go back and eliminate the fact that they didn't see you and cut you off. It already happened. It's in the past.

Did you stop them from cutting off someone else in the future? Highly unlikely. People make mistakes and will continue to do so, regardless of the consequences.

Do you know why I got cut off on my motorcycle? They didn't see me. And nothing I do now or after the fact will lead to them or anyone else seeing me better in the future, short of wearing neon colors and having flashing lights on the bike (like the police).

Sure, I can have loud pipes (I do). Doesn't always help. I could beep every time I pass or when next to someone on the road. Not sure that's practical. Haven't tried it (every time I pass someone), though I do actually use my horn as it was meant to if I recognize that I may be in a blind spot and not seen.

Common sense.

My job, as I see it, is to constantly practice awareness and get really good at knowing what's going on around me at all times. It's my responsibility to keep myself safe out there.

That's what real self defense is. Keeping safe to the best of your ability in the real world, not always staying home watching TV or looking at the four walls and avoiding life, so nothing bad happens!

So if I'm not paying attention and someone else hits me, regardless whether it's a car, bike, or I'm walking, I see it as my fault. I could have done something to avoid it. (Even leaving some space in front of me when pulling to a stop so I can pull out just in case someone comes barreling down on me because they weren't paying attention and didn't see those in front of them stopped).

That's diligence.

That's why I cannot understand how people can just put their head down and walk across a busy street without looking, whether or not they are at a crosswalk (but especially then) thinking to themselves that they have the right of way. Anything can happen.

If they get hit, the law will say they are right but does that even matter? They may also be seriously injured or even killed regardless of whose fault it is!

That's not very smart.

Please, take responsibility for your own safety. It doesn't matter who's right or wrong. What matters is the result.

So, What's More Important, the Horn or the Brake?

I once parked my car in front of a friend's house for a visit, got out and walked to the sidewalk. Out of the corner of my eye, I saw something down the road that got my attention. A car was moving toward where I had parked and appeared to be a little too close to the side where my car was.

I then watched in disbelief as it crashed right into the back of my car and then spun around ending up on the other side in front of my car. That's how hard she hit it.

The woman was okay thankfully. She explained to the police that she just took a moment to reach down and change the radio station. A simple momentary lapse in attention to the road is all it took. It could have been a lot worse.

Brings to mind all the phone calls and texting among other driver distractions. It really does only take a momentary lapse in attention.

What can you do when this happens to you? Will anger fix it?

Of course not.

The Need for Respect

You want respect? Do your absolute best in whatever you do. If you're going to do something get it done to the best of your ability. Show up when you say you're going to. Be sincere. Only you know when you're really doing your best, or not.

Be completely honest and have integrity. People should know they can trust and count on you.

No matter what.

If you're going to go through life wishy-washy and half-hearted how can you feel like you deserve respect? It doesn't matter how people treat you. Especially in today's world, where there's more smoke blown up your 'you know where' because of how thin-skinned people are. They'll pretend to respect you, but they don't.

And people want to be taken care of, instead of stepping up and being personally responsible for their lives.

Be better than that. Through practice, become strong enough to care for yourself and when someone really does need help or someone to lean on you can be there for them. Hopefully, living in this way is a positive influence that results in more self-sufficiency and better lives.

But They Don't Respect Me!

So you're upset or even angry because someone doesn't respect you. Why?

Don't say, "Because they don't respect me!" If you do, you're missing the point.

Whether you consider yourself successful or not, you have to realize if you're consistently applying yourself and sincerely doing your best, you can respect yourself.

And once you respect yourself it doesn't matter what anyone else thinks, says, or does. You know the truth for yourself. Now if they don't show you the respect you think you deserve it really is their problem, not yours.

Unless you make it yours.

You see, many times people who don't feel like they get enough respect it's really all in their own minds and imagination. They think they're not shown enough respect. It's a belief, not a fact.

The truth is other people are more focused on themselves. Everyone has their own issues. Why do we make their issues our issues?

So thinking that someone isn't showing you respect is most likely because they really aren't giving you much thought at all. They're more absorbed in what they're doing and the troubles or concerns they have. And whether or not you're showing them respect.

It's better to be passive. It's better to be centered. It's better to treat everyone as equals and with respect regardless of what they do in return.

This results in a more positive and optimistic outlook within, which has a positive influence on those around you. You're then more likely to be treated well as a result of how you naturally treat others.

But don't treat others well just because they treat you well. Treat others well anyway. No matter what. Be consistent. If it has a positive influence great. If it doesn't, that's okay too. Do it anyway.

No worries. Worry causes stress and stress kills. It makes life miserable, emotional, and leads to countless diseases. We need to apply more ways to reduce stress.

Everything we think, everything we say, and everything we do affects what we experience. Do you want those thoughts, words, and actions to be working for you or against you?

That's why you have to respect yourself first.

If you respect yourself and you love life you want a good life. You don't sit back waiting for someone else to make it better. You start with your thoughts and your words inside you.

In other words, how you talk to yourself. Are you nice to yourself? Or do you mostly tell yourself you're not worthy, you aren't good enough, or you'll never get what you really want?

Maybe you're running an old recording inside from your parents or grandparents, or a negative teacher you had or someone else who told you that crap, and you believed them. Now those same words keep repeating in your head.

Guess what? You can change those thoughts or words anytime you want. You need to respect yourself first. So plant a positive seed: the right thoughts, the right words, and then you follow it with the right actions.

"Right" meaning what? It takes you on the path you want to go. The path that should get you where you want to be in life. That's when you have direction.

That's why when you respect yourself, your time and your effort, you have some form of vision for yourself and your life. A goal for yourself maybe.

Without a goal, how can you know how to direct your thoughts, words, and deeds? You can just run around in circles, keeping busy but getting nowhere. (Unlike Ba Gua Zhang, where you would walk in circles with purpose!)

If you respect yourself, your life, and your time on this Earth, you must make some decisions and give yourself some direction so you can focus your efforts on that path. And along that path, you treat others well. Then others will more than likely treat you well in return.

This way you come from an internal influence rather than an external influence. Continually do the work on yourself. Fix what you'd like to fix, change what you'd like to change, if anything, and stop wasting time and energy and emotions trying to fix or change the outside world.

Can we apply ourselves to change the world? Sure, but first you must work on yourself.

Again, as Gandhi put it: "Be the change you wish to see in the world."

Why stress and complain about what you cannot control?

So the efforts we make to work on ourselves, to train ourselves, is what results in the real changes we experience. Ultimately, this is what gives you real freedom.

Do You Really Want Freedom?

I was discussing this with the kids in our youth Kung Fu program, and it seemed confusing to them. The look in their eyes showed that they weren't sure what I was asking.

The question was, do you prefer to be controlled by what's inside you or something or someone from the outside telling you what to do? Would you rather choose for yourself or have someone else choosing for you, determining how you feel or what you do?

Most of them started to get what I was asking, but one little boy raised his hand saying that he'd prefer someone else deciding for him. I told him that he was certainly entitled to his opinion, but I asked him, "Why?" Why would you not want to be able to make your own decisions about what you think, what you feel or what you do?

He didn't have an answer. He apparently didn't really understand.

Think about that for a moment. What is true freedom? You're free to think whatever you want. You're free to say whatever you want. You're free to do whatever you want.

It's your choice.

That's real freedom. I don't think this young boy understands the ramifications of what he was saying he wanted; to not have that choice. He was saying that he wants to be controlled by something on the outside rather than from what comes from within. If he did understand, he is saying that he wants to be controlled, told what to do, and not think for himself.

We believe that we live in a free country here in the U.S., but do we really want freedom?

The very definition of freedom is the freedom to choose what you think, say or do. Do you prefer NOT to have this freedom? There are plenty of adults who prefer not to take responsibility for themselves, want more from their government (which costs more and comes from higher taxes on those who do take responsibility for themselves).

Like the child, they don't really understand the ramifications.

When outside influences determine how you feel it shows you are controlled by the outside and not what's inside you. If you can say that you do your absolute best in all your endeavors, then do you think you deserve respect? What if you don't get it?

Respect yourself through your honest efforts, then let the outside world be whatever it is and do whatever it does.

Fear of Freedom?

I think real freedom scares people. When you're not told what to do it's up to you.

Now you're responsible, and there is no one to blame when things don't go your way.

And if you don't have some sort of vision for your life, some sort of direction, that can be a very scary thing.

It's easier if you're told what to do. Then when things don't work out, you have someone to blame and point your finger at. This takes the focus off of you, the real culprit.

So nothing changes.

I only can speak for myself, but I know what I love. I know what I'm passionate about. I find that there isn't enough time in the day for all that I'd like to do and all the things I really want to do. I wake up in the morning, and I can't wait to get started. It's that enjoyable just to be given another day to learn more, practice more, try to improve this way or that way, and to fully experience what's next in this life I'm living - in the moment, as it's happening.

It's that much fun because I have that freedom. What can be more valuable than being able to get up in the morning and do what you love to do with your day?

That's why if you hate your job and you're miserable in your relationship, you have to re-evaluate. You have to ask yourself, "Why?"

Why do you hate your job? Is it really the job? Have you ever loved any job?

Or is it you'd rather be spending your time doing someone else?

If you don't know yourself, it's very difficult to answer that question.

The same can be said for relationships. Why do so many marriages end up in divorce?

These two people loved each other at one point, that's why they got married! However, somewhere along the line, they forgot. They stopped trying. They stopped caring for each other. They stopped showing each other the attention that they once did which got them connected in the beginning.

If you can sit back and calm the mind, getting rid of all the head trash, and go back to look and remember why you fell in love in the first place it all becomes clear. Then you may want to make an effort again because you realize it's worth it.

People do change. Sometimes there is nothing you can do about it and moving on is the best option. However, the grass isn't always greener... somewhere, or with someone, else.

Your Perspective in Life

How you see things determines what you experience. Who's in control of you? How you see things; what you say to yourself; showing respect regardless of what others do in return; etc. Is it family, religion, cultural background, media, or something else?

Is respect really about the other person?

When I enter the training area of our school (dojang, dojo) and no one is around, I still bow and salute. My teacher is not there to accept my respect. It cannot make him feel respected. So, who is it for?

It's for me, of course.

My mind is full of gratitude. I'm grateful for what I've learned and where it came from. I'm grateful and appreciate that I have this space to train and do the work on myself and to share with others on the same path.

And that feels good inside.

If I bow and salute to a student and see them as another spark of the Divine, I get a wonderful feeling inside of me.

Guess what happens inside you when you feel good: Your body relaxes; Qi and blood flow smoothly throughout your body; you feel more positive and optimistic which brings more good thoughts; you're happier, healthier, and enjoy your life more.

You feel more peaceful and less emotional.

That's why I see respect completely from the other side. It's for my benefit to respect others. It improves a relationship, so I benefit. It allows me to learn from the other person, rather than always thinking "I'm better" and "Let me tell you what I know..." So again, I benefit.

Having respect, from this perspective, sets my mind right to learn and enjoy life more.

Meditation and Perspective

The consistent practice of meditation allows you to get a deep sense of self, a clear awareness of your thoughts and the ability to control those thoughts. You cannot control what you're not aware of.

With a calmer mind, outside influences don't have much effect on you.

So if you respect yourself, your life and your time, this practice and the time you spend working on yourself, including your time in meditation, is the most important thing you can do every day for a better future.

My Dear Old Dad

When my father was in his mid-fifties, just a few years older than I am as I write this, he was already breaking down physically. He had bad knees as long as I can remember. He didn't exercise and ate whatever he wanted but took a variety of vitamins and other over-the-counter pills recommended in all sorts of ads and magazine articles.

He had no real guidance from a trained professional and even if he did go to see one and was advised to change his SAD

(Standard American Diet) dietary habits he would argue and ultimately ignore them. No one was going to be taking away his pizza!

It wasn't long before he was diagnosed with prostate cancer.

Long story short, he opted for a hormone injection known as Lupron to shrink the prostate and control the cancer. Every time he received this shot he would feel weaker in his legs until one day he was so weak he missed his bed when trying to sit and broke his hip when he fell.

He never walked again and lived the last three years of his life in bed. He was basically a quadriplegic and needed round-the-clock care. He lived in a few nursing homes before finally being brought home to live out his last days more comfortably, cared for mostly by my mother and daily visits from nurses. He degenerated quickly in this condition. It was painful to watch.

If you research just this one treatment (there are so many) you will find seemingly endless lies and corruption:

"At least one expert believes Lupron should be pulled from the market. Dr. John L. Gueriguian, a former medical officer with the US Food and Drug Administration (FDA), stated in a report for a pharmaceutical liability lawsuit on 3/19/08 that Lupron should not be used."

"After years of use of [Lupron] in a great number of patients, the evidence is clear that TAP [Takeda Abbott Pharmaceuticals] didn't study [Lupron] adequately before marketing," Gueriguian states in his report. "After its introduction into the marketplace, TAP did not perform enough long-term studies to detect potential long-term and irreversible side effects of [Lupron], which has been shown, through independent observations and studies, to be able to cause irreversible side effects and permanent severely disabling health problems. Lupron temporarily stops menstruation but does not eradicate endometriosis for long-term. Lupron should only be limited to six injections for the initial treatment, and a retreatment should not exceed six injections. Lupron cannot be given more than twelve injections per lifetime."

[Source: bit.ly/lupron-risks]

My father received this shot every three months for twelve years. That's forty-eight shots, *four times the recommended lifetime limit!*

But that's another story...

The point here is:

1. I don't want to age like that (so I will do the opposite), and
2. Short of an accident or trauma of some kind that alters one's body structurally, our day-by-day and moment-by-moment decisions determine our health.

Watching my father's unnecessary demise is motivation enough to do whatever I can, as well as teach others the same, so any *perceived need* to seek dangerous pharmaceutical drugs to hide symptoms (your body's only way to talk to you and ask for change) can be avoided.

Follow Success...

If someone is where I want to be and they are willing to show me how they got there, all I have to do is put my head down and walk the same path.

No sense being pig-headed and stuck on a path that just isn't working. Regardless of how you got there, adjust!

This has helped me to keep improving my body (strength and mobility) and my mind (better mental attitude and more emotional stability). Even as I have now reached my fifties, I still experience improvement physically. Sure, recovery time isn't what it used to be, but being smart and only doing the right amount of physical training by listening to what my body is telling me, the improvements continue every year.

For some this is impossible. When corrected, these people feel somehow inferior, picked on, or just feel like they'll *never* get it. So eventually, they give up and let father time beat them down.

We have to be better than that. We can be better than that.

Instead, get excited when someone who has already walked the path you are on and found success reaches out to help and points out flaws in your approach. This is an opportunity for growth, not judgment. See it as clear direction giving you something to focus on.

Not having something to focus on is what leads to boredom.

If you know where you want to go and someone who's been there can point the way, why fight it? Why think you can come up with a better way? Just go!

After you've successfully reached whatever goal you've set for yourself and can look back at the path from a place of real knowledge and experience, and believe that you have a better way based on having traveled the path for yourself, then and only then should you speak of it.

Following the path that's already been laid out by others before you is not weak or an inferior approach, it is a wise approach and saves you time. Then you can "get there" faster, leaving more time to go even further.

If every generation had to reinvent the wheel because it was kept secret by those who came before, then you can be sure we wouldn't all be driving around in cars today.

Every generation builds on the success of the previous one as long as there is open and honest sharing instead of holding back "secrets" due solely to self-interest and the profit motive.

What You Believe and What Actually Works

Sometimes when making recommendations for a patient in my clinic, we may come across an area where there is some fundamental disagreement. It may be religious based. It may be cultural such as: "I'm Italian, I have to have my pasta!" So advising against eating it, usually meets with resistance, even if that pasta may be contributing to their ill-health.

On the one side, we have our beliefs. On the other, we have what works. If what actually works is in conflict with your beliefs, you need to rethink your beliefs if you want optimal results.

There are so many different cultures, many different ways people are brought up, many different religions, and so on. Sometimes what you *think* is true, what you've *been told* is true, *is not true at all.*

In fact, in some ways, it may be bringing you harm.

Again, the Chinese martial art, Ba Gua Zhang, is based on Daoist philosophical ideas. "Ba Gua," the "Eight Trigrams" is a Daoist concept originating in one of the oldest books known, the Yi Jing (I Ching). Dao had also been spelled "Tao," just in case you're not familiar with it. It just depends which system of Romanization one is using because it's actually a Chinese character.

The Dao has been translated as the way, the path, the road, and then some people loosely say whatever path you are on is your Dao. That's being very loose about the meaning. Originally, it was referring to the natural way, the way of nature, or what is most in line with the natural world, and that's how I am referring to it. Just simply what works, naturally.

However, because we're so smart, we think about how we can make it better, and we don't always make it better do we? We overthink things, and we create beliefs, and those beliefs can take us away from what actually works. Away from our true nature and the natural ways.

My teacher, Grandmaster Park, was very interesting in the ways he taught. Once you understand the natural laws, it becomes like a litmus test. You can ask in most any situation, "Does this make sense according to natural laws?" You know, simple things like the shortest distance between two points is a straight line. Nobody can argue. Well, I guess one *could* argue, but they'd be wrong.

No matter how many ways you want to try, the shortest distance is a straight line. It's things like that. The sun rises in the east - natural law. We can't argue with that. It doesn't matter how strongly you want to believe that it rises in the west, unless we're simply changing labels, you'd be wrong. The sun will rise from the direction it rises. California will never greet a new day before New York.

The natural world doesn't think about things so much. All life in the natural world flows with nature. If not, it struggles more and dies.

When it's warm, beings in the natural world come out. When it's cold, they find shelter. Very simple. They don't have to think about "Am I cold? Do I need a jacket?" They just feel uncomfortable, and they go find something more comfortable. Very simple, not a lot of thought there. They feel hungry, they go find something to eat. Maybe they have to hunt something, maybe they have to eat some wild edibles. But they don't sit there and get bored, and have to eat. Their body tells them when to eat, so they listen. They just eat what they need. Hungry, eat. Not hungry, do something else. Maybe nothing, just sitting still.

Grandmaster Park would talk about when he'd be asked a question. Maybe someone would say, "What about this, Shifu? What about that, Shifu?" and the student would give him some idea he'd have or something from a book somewhere because we're really good with books. We tend to think once it's written in a book, it's true. This person who wrote this must be an expert.

There are plenty of people writing books. There are plenty of people writing blogs on the internet. It doesn't make what they have to say true or accurate. It's just their opinion. It may be valid, it may be invalid.

So my Shifu would listen and say, *"This your thinking."* What does that mean, "This your thinking"?

"This not right, this your thinking." So he would teach us not to get in the way of natural principles. Don't let your intellect screw up your understanding of what's real and what's true. That is the Daoist way. Another very powerful concept in the Daoist way is recognizing one's True Self.

Imagine using a circle to represent your Original Self and then you've got a bunch of scribbles (representing noise) on top of it: all you've learned since you were born, the habits, beliefs, and reactions of your parents, your religion, your culture, etc. This is all programming. The Daoist Way would be to recognize it and clean it all away. Gradually you would purify yourself and get back to who you really are, beyond all the programming.

Now, what does that mean?

Our True Selves are just consciousness, and everything else is on top of that pure consciousness.

In class, I've used the example of a clear blue sky. When the clouds come, you don't see the clear blue sky, but it's still there. We just need the clouds to clear away so we can see it.

Most people don't even realize where all these thoughts came from. In today's world with 30, 40, 50,000 messages hitting us every day, we don't even know what our own thoughts are anymore. There's the mainstream thinking that people think is the truth. There are plenty of myths that people think are true. They do not work, but people still do them anyway. And a lot of it comes from highly educated people: doctors, PhDs, etc. They're so trained in a particular way, and they spend so much money to get their credentials, that if it is wrong, where does that leave them? They feel like they don't even know who they are anymore.

So they will fight it, to protect and keep the status quo, even if it's clearly wrong. Historically, how many died for someone to maintain what they believed to be true? How many wars were fought throughout human history because people had to make sure to maintain that, "Our way is the right way and their way cannot be?"

"That can't be right because it's not our way. And if they're right, that makes us wrong. We can't be wrong! So let's kill them, take their land, and make our way the only way."

The only true way is the natural way and anything that has something different than that cannot be the right way. In nature, there really is only one way. You survive! You eat, you get shelter, you drink water, you breathe the air, you get the sunlight - that's the simple way. Everything else, we added to it. What kind of house is better? What kind of religion is better? What kind of money is better? What kind of car is better? What makes me look better? We made it more and more complicated than ever. And mine is better than yours. And if someone else's is better, maybe you want to take theirs.

The Gods Must Be Crazy

That reminds me, a long time ago I saw a movie. It's an old movie, "The Gods Must Be Crazy," where a group of native Bushmen are living in perfect harmony, all happy and laughing with each other, enjoying things, sharing everything and going about their daily lives. A plane comes by, and the pilot throws an empty soda bottle right out the window.

The narrator describes the scene from the perspective of the Bushmen of the Kalahari, people living in harmony with nature, as they have since the beginning of time:

... *"But in the Kalahari, it's always Tuesday, or Thursday if you like. Or Sunday. No clocks or calendars tell you to do this or that.*

Lately, strange new things sometimes appeared in the sky. Noisy birds that flew without flapping their wings.

One day, something fell from the sky. Xi had never seen anything like this in his life. It looked like water, but it was harder than anything else in the world. He wondered why the gods had sent this thing down to the earth. It was the strangest and most beautiful thing they had ever seen.

They wondered why the gods had sent it to them. Pabo got his finger stuck in the thing and the children thought he was very funny. Xi tried the thing out to cure thongs. It had the right shape and weight.

It was also beautifully smooth and ideal for curing snakeskin. And Pabo discovered you could make music on it. And every day they discovered a new use for the thing. It was harder and heavier and smoother than anything they'd ever known. It was the most useful thing the gods had ever given them. A real labor-saving device.

But the gods had been careless. They had sent only one.

Now, for the first time, here was a thing that could not be shared because there was only one of it. Suddenly, everybody needed it most of the time. A thing they had never needed before became a necessity. And unfamiliar emotions began to stir. A feeling of wanting to own, of not wanting to share. Other new things came: anger, jealousy, hate and violence."

They were all in perfect harmony when everything belonged to everyone. But all of a sudden, there was this one special thing, and it screwed them all up. You see, native people only knew the natural way. They lived a simple life in accordance with the Dao.

So do we have to go back to the native ways, live the way they do, wear the same clothes and eat the same foods?

That's not the point. What's important here is what's going on in your head? How purely can you go back to natural thinking and how can you side-step your beliefs, especially if they're not working for you?

I believe in one way, the way of nature. Our practice, which must include meditation, can make whatever religious or spiritual beliefs you have stronger. You get more connected to the Divine, God, the Creator, the Source. You can experience a "direct-connect" all on your own.

What I have a problem with is when a religion thinks that their way is the only way. Because if your religion is right and people who don't believe in that religion are going to Hell, isn't that strange? This one believes they're right, another believes they're right, and yet another one believes they're right. Who's right? All of them or none of them. Think about it.

The Daoist way is to step away from all of that. Just let everyone be, having their own experience. Our practice should help us get to that point of living in peace. Peace within and peace without. Stop the fighting on the outside with others and on the inside with yourself. Watch what you say especially to yourself. Be nice to yourself.

Experiencing the Results of Your Beliefs

Do your beliefs lead to poor health? Do your beliefs lead to more stress? Do your beliefs lead to more peace or more conflict? We can take a good look at that. If we live a little more consciously, we can take a good look at that and if we don't like the results we're getting we can say, maybe this path, these beliefs aren't so good.

When I think my way is the right way, then I get pissed off when someone isn't living in a similar or consistent way, that causes me stress. And if I start arguing and getting on someone else's case, that creates stress for them, too. Which is basically spreading negativity and difficulty, creating more suffering.

The Daoist way is non-judgmental. The goal in life is to purify your mind, figure out who you really are and get back to your True Nature. Then try to live closest to that.

How far can you go without labeling things? When we label, we attach our own baggage. It's what we *think* we know about something or someone. This limits and also propagates our programming, making it very difficult to experience anything as it truly is.

I know my parents' generation, it's a common practice to figure out how they can label you. You know, "the white boy, the Jewish kid, the Muslim, black people, brown people, red people, purple people (or whatever)." Then we somehow think we know them better because of it. "Ah, that's the druggie. She's trouble." (You might not say any of these out loud, but in your thoughts...). If you play sports are you automatically a good guy?

What if you meet a martial artist? What does that bring to mind? An MMA "human cock-fighter" or the old master of peace?

Labels. Can you see through the labels? How far can you go without using them?

Not Just Punching and Kicking

A goal of mine is to help more people to realize that this practice is so much more than punching and kicking. We master our body through use. We make good circulation through our body through using the four limbs. We get our mind clear by meditation. We relax the body and mind through breathing. And then we feel better, more optimistic, more positive, and we treat others better, too.

We have a practice that brings more peace within so we can have more peace around us, instead of judgment and conflict. That is the Daoist way - to live in harmony.

Back to the question and a quick review: You have your beliefs and you have what works. Do your beliefs conflict with what works? If so, you need to rethink your beliefs.

CHAPTER 28

The Blind Men and the Elephant

Have you heard the story of the blind men who come upon an elephant, each with a unique perspective describing what they think is an accurate depiction of an elephant?

One describes the elephant as a wall, "It's a big wall!"

Another one says, "No, it's like a big tree trunk. The elephant is like a tree trunk."

Another one, "No, it's a branch. Look, I can hang on it."

And the last, "It's more like a snake. It's thin and moves around."

Of course, they're all wrong because someone who can see walks up and sees the whole thing, the big picture, with one glance, and can tell them, "No, you're only seeing from where you are, your perspective."

And let's not forget the fact that they're actually blind. We never consider ourselves blind because we can see. But can we? As I said earlier, I like to put it this way, "We don't see things as they are, we see things as we think they are."

If you put five people in a traumatic situation, not only will you have five different descriptions of what happened, you can have five very different reactions.

One might end up in therapy. Another one might end up teaching others about it. Another one may become stronger, another one becomes crushed. One learns what he can do, another one what he (thinks he) can't do.

All from the same experience.

I can't tell you how many times I've come across people, patients, or students, who explain to me why they're so stressed. It's their job, their family, their kids, they're always looking outside of themselves.

If I share what I see from my perspective, that it all comes from inside and depends on how they see things, what I see in their eyes is that they don't get it because they believe it's just their life and there's nothing they can do about it.

Now, it's true. You could be in a really difficult situation. However, some people respond one way, some people respond another way. How do you respond? Because that is ultimately what's going to determine what you do next or what you experience because of it. The same situation can lead to different experiences depending on the person's beliefs and perspective.

So remember the blind men, each from their own angle, and then think about how you may be blind one way or another. Is it your religious background? Is it your cultural background? Is it your parents' teaching? Is it what you learned in school?

You know, a kid grows up with an alcoholic father who beats the mother compared to another kid whose father is like his best friend, the two people have a very different view of what a father is. Can you see that? Because depending on how you grew up, that's how your brain literally developed. That's how your perspective literally developed and has determined how you see the world.

Many years ago, this really came to light for me because of the title, "Shifu"...

The Meaning of "Shifu"

"Shi" (师, sounds like "shr") is defined as, "teacher," "master," or "specialist." It can also mean, "model; example." "Fu" (父) literally means, "father." So it's like saying, "teacher-father."

It can be used to address the head of a Chinese martial arts school, or dojang. Historically, many orphans were taken in by old Kung Fu masters and taught how to live in the world and to have a better life. So the master was very much like a father.

In the Japanese dojo, they use "Sensei."

"Sensei" translates literally as "person born before" and means that they are "further down the road". Again, this is like a father, (or older brother/sister). So after you've been down the road, you know where the obstacles are, you know where the various potholes are, and you can help others avoid those things along the way. You have the knowledge and experience acquired along that road. On the other hand, when you're the pilgrim, or the first one down the path, everything is brand new. Then you can easily fall into every trap and be held up by every obstacle.

So, the Sensei can lead others by experience. This "father," as discussed above, is supposed to be just like your parent. He's supposed to have gone through life ahead of you, and should be able to provide proper guidance in life.

However, what's the father's perspective? If the father's perspective is all twisted, then they're going to have a twisted perspective that they teach the child as well. That's why I take that term and position to heart. To me, it's a constant reminder; an ideal to live up to every day.

My teachers in my life, my mentors in my life, they helped make me who I am. Doing my best every day is a way of paying homage to them. It's an ideal. It's not a pedestal. It's not a "better than" attitude at all. If anything, it's a responsibility.

And it's not easy.

But the problem was, "Shifu" meaning "teacher-father" and the person who grew up with a horrible father or a father who left them when they were a child or some other bad experience with a father figure in their life. Their father brings back terrible memories of abuse or neglect. Then they learn that "Shifu" can be equated with "father" and it doesn't sit well with them at all. They may understandably react negatively thinking, "I don't want any part of this."

We each have our own perspective. But that's the same as thinking all men (or women) are bad. All white people (or black, or brown, or Hispanic, etc.) are bad. All Muslims (or Jews, or Christians, or Hindus, etc.) are bad. We think we know, but we don't.

I think you get the point.

You see, my perspective of "Shifu" is an ideal to strive for. Their perspective of a father is completely different. So they get a bad feeling from it. I have a good feeling from it. Heck, their bad experience could have been with a martial arts instructor, or it could have been a dance instructor.

There was a well-liked local dance instructor in the next town over from our dojang a few years back who was turned in for multiple accounts of molesting children. Now imagine that's your experience with a Shifu or Sensei. You learn or experience that Shifu is molesting children. You go through that, and the title disgusts you. You'd have a very negative perspective of what a Shifu is.

I am sorry for what others do with their positions. But that has nothing to do with me.

Personally, I take the title and role very seriously. It is a constant reminder of what an impact I can have (both positive and negative) by example. My experience has been very positive, and every day I work to pay forward for future generations what I was fortunate enough to have learned from my teachers, mentors, and my Shifu.

I know it can change lives.

There are varying viewpoints on using the term, or title, "Shifu." To some, it is a sort of bastardization by American teachers and in bad taste. However, my experience and opinion differ from theirs, and I am not concerned with their view of what is or is not appropriate.

Ironically, you'll even hear it used regularly in old Chinese language Kung Fu movies. They are referring to their teacher as "master," which is one of the meanings for the term, as is "a person of skill."

For me, it is very special, even sacred, and not a pedestal but a responsibility. It is a title that must be continuously earned, in my opinion.

Although I have observed it used beyond martial arts (my acupuncture teacher was also called, "Shifu" by his closest students, who were indeed Chinese), and *Laoshi* may be considered more correct to many, as my own Shifu described it: It is more personal and "like family." Whereas "laoshi" is more academic.

I've used both to address various Chinese martial arts teachers from China. So, it really is what you make of it.

An interesting aside I'd like to share here (from https://www.med.uottawa.ca/sim/data/Physician_e.htm):

"The word, "doctor" means teacher, from the Latin docere, "to teach."

The word, "physician" means "naturalist," from the Greek word for nature (physis; physikos meant "natural"). Many medicines were, of course, derived from natural substances, and in early language "physic" referred to medicines."

It is not much of a stretch to see that the doctors and physicians of ancient times could also be called "Shifu," as they were the ones teaching people how to live in harmony with natural ways and to be healthy.

Basic Civility

In the not too distant past, knowing someone on a first name basis meant you were close, and your relationship was more personal with them. Referring to someone by their first name assumes this.

Nowadays people do it regardless of their relationship and assume this closeness without having earned it or by being granted any permission to cross that line from formal to personal by the person they are addressing.

Here a certain purity and even civility are in order to maintain the most advantageous relationship conducive to learning.

Maintaining titles and not crossing certain lines when addressing teachers keeps the teacher-student relationship intact.

This is especially important for the student and matters little, if at all, to the teacher.

For example, I address my teacher of Chinese medicine as, "Dr. Zhang." However, there are many who also learn from him that call him, "Jimmy." I find this disrespectful and even a hindrance to learning.

When you make a great teacher out to be like your buddy, you bring him or her down to your level and to "feel equal." But they are not your equal. They have more knowledge and experience. Isn't that why you choose to learn from them?

It is my opinion that addressing a teacher properly allows me to maintain a higher level of respect and even reverence for their level of experience and their teaching. It enhances my ability to learn from that person. There are subconscious psychological effects at work here that can work for you or against you.

I don't need to be my teacher's buddy. We are friendly, but not friends.

I have witnessed the problems with this attitude numerous times in my years. Familiarity breeds contempt. The teacher, who is seen as a friend or buddy, is more likely to be argued with. This can greatly hinder the learning process.

And the student is the one who loses.

In my opinion, it is for the same reason, as stated earlier, that even when alone in my martial arts school I will bow and salute when I enter the training area with respect for my teacher and all who came before me as well as gratitude in my heart for the special space and opportunity to practice. That is for me.

Remember, *I am alone.* My teacher is not there to enjoy or acknowledge my salute and respect.

A story told by long-time strength and conditioning specialist, Dan John, in his book, "Never Let Go" helps to further express and maybe better clarify my perspective:

"I never wanted to be a coach, but everybody calls me Coach. I remember shuddering when I heard Coach referring to me, yet now I embrace it. My attitude changed a few years ago when I met a man named Coach. We met at a conference and he had taken voluminous notes from my talk. He came up afterwards and waited patiently while I answered the usual questions about all the things I didn't talk about during the lecture. Generally, if I don't talk about something, it is because I don't think it is important. He excused himself and asked for some clarification about a few small items."

"I asked him his name and he said, "Coach."

"Fine," I said, "but what's your name?"

His answer changed my life. "When I was a young man, I was a terror. I did all the wrong things and I knew I was doing wrong. At the local community center, I started playing some ball. There was a man there who took no nonsense from me. He expected more. He demanded more. The man turned my life around. And, as soon as I could, I decided to dedicate my life to his memory. All I know of him is that we called him Coach. Please, all I ever want to be, and all I ever want to be known as is Coach. Call me Coach."

"Call me Coach."

I feel the same about what traditional martial arts and my Shifu have meant to my life. My character and perspective has been shaped by my experiences with more than one of these teachers. They were examples for me to follow. If I can be that for someone else and be even a small part of helping to make even one life better, it would be an honor and a privilege.

Again, it's a responsibility and a constant reminder of an ideal I want to live up to every day. I've dedicated my life to pass on what I received from them so that the next generation and beyond will benefit the same.

My teacher called his teacher Shifu. I called my teacher Shifu.

Call me Shifu.

Your Perspective Determines Your Experience

So now, turn that into other things in your life. Your perspective of things, your perspective of your position in the world. It's like Henry Ford said, "Whether you think you can or think you can't, you're right." That's perspective.

Some people can try anything in life and have no concern for failure. They just try, and they fail, and they try again, and they fail again. In fact, some of the most successful people on this planet have failed more than anybody else.

Think again of Babe Ruth. As discussed earlier in the chapter on Perseverance, they say he was the strikeout king. Most don't know that because he's known for the home runs. Every time he got up he was swinging for the fences. And when you swing that hard, you strikeout a lot. He wasn't worried about striking out.

Many baseball players focus on just hitting the ball for singles. That's a lot easier. But the fans came to see Babe Ruth hit home runs. When he got up, he'd swing, and most of the time he'd make an out. But when they saw that home run, everybody would get up and cheer the loudest. That's what Babe lived for.

Other people never even want to step to the plate. They never even want to try. Why? Maybe something in their life as a child raising their hand and coming up with an idea and everybody laughed. And they never forgot that. One time, scarred for life. So now they're deathly afraid of ever having to speak in front of anybody, and they don't want to ever run into people that they went to school with because it's such a bad experience in their world and in their life.

And so, that person always thinks they can't because trying something, stepping up in front of others, is this threat of repeating that horrible feeling.

To me, the practice of martial arts is about overcoming these limitations that we put on ourselves. It's about realizing how we're blind. It's about getting over our beliefs and changing our perspective and starting to clear the way for "who am I really?"

I'm not simply the person who's been scarred or whose life is run by those experiences, positive or negative. But it's a heck of a lot better, and life is a lot more fun if you come up willing to try things and not worry about failing, and more optimistic than pessimistic about how things might go.

There is No Bravery Without Fear

Those who are brave enough to face their fears are constantly trying and experiencing new things, so they always have new experiences to draw on. They enjoy a growing and expanding world. If you are like this, then the world is your oyster.

Those who run from their fears and let fear run them are always avoiding anything new or uncomfortable, so they never grow beyond their current comfort zone. They miss out on so much of what life has to offer. They experience a shrinking world, and the world is their prison.

As previously discussed in Chapter 4, we fear what we don't know or understand. It is one thing to jump in head first to face your fears, no matter what, but with a little preparation and accumulation of knowledge, we can develop the courage necessary to succeed when facing a challenge.

Courage and bravery are not the same. To have courage, you must first understand what it is you are facing. Any empty-headed moron, who has no concept of the danger he's exposing himself to, (and maybe others, as well), can fearlessly run into a fire, (or any equivalent), and get himself, (and/or others) killed. That may seem brave, but again, there is no bravery without fear.

Acquiring the necessary skills and knowledge to be better prepared for a surprise allows you to make a wiser decision.

That's courage.

Having the wherewithal to throw dirt in the eyes of a hungry tiger, who's moving in on you for the kill, is bravery. Whereas running away, (or freezing) gives you no chance at all. Just having considered that seemingly impossible situation is preparation. This allows you to "keep thinking," so a possible solution can be realized in an emergency.

Bravery without courage is short-lived. It has no real root and can quickly run out of steam. Think of an ancient battlefield, where the leaders get their military to yell and scream in order to build them up in the face of death.

Once these men see those around them getting killed, without proper preparation and developed skills, their fear will take over. They will most likely freeze and then lose their lives because they are unable to fight.

Just as well, if they forge ahead and still do not have adequate preparation and skills, they will also quickly lose their life when facing those who are better prepared.

So many allow fear to run them. If there is something that you want to get done or accomplished, the first step to having the courage to do it is to make sure you understand what it is going to take to get it done, as well as what it is that you are afraid of.

A valid fear can save your life, just as bravery can get you killed. That's why courage is actually what you need first.

Courage comes from knowledge. Knowledge is power, but knowledge without action is nothing.

That's where bravery comes in. You actually have to step up and do what needs to be done when the time comes. If you know what to do, then all you need is be brave in the moment.

With worry and fear your world gets smaller, more limited, and stressful.

Let that go.

With courage and bravery your world gets bigger, feels limitless, and more joyful.

Embrace it.

Are You the Optimist or the Pessimist?

Things never work out for the pessimist, you know. They're always looking for, and so seeing, the worst.

The optimist sees every failure as one step closer to success.

Pessimists - every failure is, "See? I can't do it!" And they tend to see the negative in things.

Ask yourself: "Do I focus on the good or do I focus on the bad? Am I an optimist or a pessimist? Do I dwell on my troubles?"

Focus on what is wrong or bad and you will find it. This leads to constant frustration. Successful people focus on what is right and good. What seems like trouble today, can be a blessing tomorrow.

Good News, Bad News, Who Knows?

There once was a farmer who owned a beautiful horse. One day, during a great storm, the horse was spooked and broke out of his stall.

A neighbor came by to console him saying, "Oh what bad news to have lost such a beautiful horse."

The farmer shrugged and said only, "Good news, bad news, who knows?"

The horse returned a few days later with three other beautiful horses. The neighbor came by to proclaim the good news but the farmer said only, "Good news, bad news, who knows?"

Soon after, the farmer's eighteen-year-old son broke his leg while trying to ride one of the wild horses, and of course the neighbor came by and said, "Oh, such terrible news that your son has broken his leg. I'm so sorry for you."

But the farmer only said, "Good news, bad news, who knows?"

Then the military came through looking to bring all the young able-bodied men that could find into the war, but the farmer's son was of no use with a broken leg.

Good news, bad news... who really knows? Which one would you rather be? Which attitude would you rather have? And if you're a parent, what do you want to teach your children?

So when the parents have a problem, they put it on the children, and then the children end up with the same problem, or way of thinking. So what are genetic problems, really? Are they really just habits passed down from generation to generation?

If you eat pretty much the same kind of food and have most of the same hang-ups and issues, essentially seeing the world in the same way, because the parents raise the children with their beliefs and perspective of the world, you're going to end up with a very similar experience mentally, emotionally, with your health, etc.

If you're afraid of bugs and you scream every time there's a bug, the child learns to be afraid of bugs. But if the parents get down and play with the bugs, then the children want to play with the bugs. It's an ignorance-based fear.

If you know whether they're poisonous or dangerous in any way, then you know whether to avoid or ignore. We assume they're a threat because we don't understand (and they tend to be ugly!). So if you have a fear of bugs or snakes or anything else, educate yourself about what's dangerous and what's not. Then you will know.

At home, we have reptiles, and some of them eat crickets. So, we always have a big bin of crickets. Crickets are pretty cool actually. They're funny if you give them a chance. Do you know you can make a friend with a cricket? Yes, you can make friends with a cricket. I'll bet you didn't know that.

I've done it while lying out on the grass outside my home. Because as with any animal, if you're calm, and you're not threatening, they learn to trust you. It's very interesting. I've had a cricket in my hand sitting out in the grass for, you know, 10, 15, 20 minutes, until I was done with it.

Then I'd eat 'em.

Just kidding.

It was on my hand, on my finger. It doesn't jump away. But if you try to get it, if you do something threatening, then it will get nervous and try to flee.

Most people see the cricket bin, and they respond along the lines of, "Ahh!!! Bugs!" It's so funny. My kids were like that early on, too. But I'd put my hand in there, and they can all crawl on my hand, it's absolutely safe. They don't bite. There's nothing to it. It's a funny thing to experience.

And in their own way, they're cute. But I digress...

Are Your Fears Valid?

So what are you afraid of, and why do you think it's valid? Do you live your life in a way that reflects those fears?

People tend to think things such as: when my husband acts the way I want him to, when my children do as they're told, when my job is what I want it to be - then I'll be happy, then I'll feel better, then I won't be sick, then I won't be stressed. But because of (fill in the blank) I'm stressed.

Remember, we don't see things as they are. We see things as we think they are, and we usually want them to be different. So the perspective of acceptance that the world is the world, it is what it is, and I have to live in the world, the world is not there for me alone, it's not going to change just for me. My experience of it just depends on how I see things. Then how I respond to those things.

Does it make me happy? Does it make me sick? Same world.

Learn to see things as they are. That's where meditation comes in. To clear the mind of all our B.S. and see people as they are, see your children as they are, see the job as it is.

Maybe it really is a problem. If so, you can change. But the easier thing - I don't know how easy, but you have this choice. You have the option to change your expectations.

Dead, but Still Breathing

How many marriages break up and end in divorce? Two people love each other, at least they think they do, they get married, and it's supposed to be 'till death do us part, but that death comes much earlier than expected? You know, their body is still alive, they're still breathing, but the death of the person inside because they're trying to be someone they're not.

Many times, people get married and thought they married one person when they're actually a very different kind of person. And now they go through years and years, stressing over "You need to be this way. You're my wife. You're supposed to be... (however you think a wife is supposed to be)."

But they want to be the way *they* want to be. Or, simply are what they are and don't care to change.

"But I want you to be like this."

"But I'm not like that."

"But you have to be this..." and they just keep fighting over wanting to make the other person become something different then what they are.

That's stressful.

Change your expectations and find a way to accept them as they really are because there's a really good chance in the early part of the game, you didn't see them as they really were. The signs were there, but you overlooked them, didn't want to see them, or just missed them because you focused on what you loved about them.

You had this delusion, this ideal, and then when you got to know them well, everything changed. So it's the death to that person who you *thought* you were marrying. Or it's your death as you try and try to be something you're not.

It's death to those ending in divorce. It's supposed to be when the body dies, right?

Take a good look at your life.

How many things are in your life that stress you out? How many things give you problems, or make life difficult for you? Look in the mirror and ask yourself, what in your life can you change your expectations about that would make your experience of it different?

Can you accept things as they are? Can you accept the people in your life as they are, without trying to change them into something they're not?

If you can, your whole experience will change too.

Whether it's parents raising children, employer-employee, husband-wife, brother, sister, father, son, mother, daughter, are you willing to change your perspective in order to make your life better?

Or are you going to keep pounding your head against the wall and thinking one day it's not going to hurt?

You remember the definition of insanity, right? You keep doing the same thing, expecting different results.

It's much easier, and this is true Daoism: accept the world as it is, let it be, let it go, and change your expectations so you can live in peace. You can live in harmony instead of always butting heads with everything and everyone.

Remember, the blind men and the elephant. From where are you standing that you think is right?

Practicing Gratitude, Love, and Compassion

When facing all the many forms of adversity we all face, we can focus on the problems and let worry, fear and stress run our lives. Another approach is practicing gratitude.

When you feel negative, when you feel down, think of what you have.

Here is a daily habit we can all strive to have: At the end of every day when you turn the lights out, and you're ready to sleep, visualize your day. Imagine what happened throughout the day, from the moment you got up, all the way through that day, and find all the good things that happened.

We tend to be like the news. We have a habit of focusing on the bad things, and we don't even realize we're doing it. But when you actively focus on the good things that happened, you start to smile. You start to feel better, and it's easier to go to sleep in peace and with a smile on your face.

Rather than stressed and worrying about, "Oh, I can't believe he said that to me today," or what so-and-so did to you, etc.

All it takes is one little thing. It could have been someone giving you the bird on the road, and that one little thing that someone did on your way to work, then while at your job you complained to people for three hours about what happened to you on the road.

Think about how you carry these things. They gave you the bird. Instead of getting angry and taking that poison all day, have compassion. I guarantee their life is painful. If someone wants to do that to you, they want to try to give you pain, they want to yell at you, that's their problem. Leave it in their car and focus on the good things.

This keeps you in control of your inner world.

There is far too much "us against them" in this world. Truth is, we're all in this together. If we destroy the planet, we all suffer. If you hate your neighbor, you both can suffer, but mostly it's you. You're the one with the hate inside.

And as I've already said earlier, jealousy is the ugliest emotion.

If someone is doing well, we should all be uplifted and inspired. Why do so many feel the need to knock someone off their pedestal? As a society, we seem to relish in people's bad news. Jeez, just look at the tabloids (and how much money they make)!

Here's a challenge for you:

The next time you realize you're thinking badly about someone, shift your focus and see them as another spark of the Divine - just like you. Feel love in your heart for them. And have compassion for them because you know they struggle.

This may be hard to swallow, but in your heart, you can even have love and compassion for those we see as our enemies. Even the lunatics who go on shooting rampages or drive trucks through crowds of innocent people - *in your heart, you can have compassion for them.*

Accept that they are sick. What they do on the outside is a reflection of the suffering they feel on the inside. When someone is full of hate, there is no peace.

I assure you, they suffer every day.

Instead of putting so much energy into emotions like hate and fear let's focus on what we can do about it. Let's focus on how to protect ourselves and keep ourselves safe. (More on this in later chapters "The Reality of Self Defense" and "Situational Awareness...")

Now don't get me wrong, when one of these crazy people lose their lives due to decisions to hurt others so be it. If someone means to do me harm, I'm going to do whatever it takes and whatever is required to protect and defend myself.

Hopefully, no more than is necessary.

If they're hurt, I will offer help in any way that I can. There will be no anger going forward. I have no interest in carrying that baggage. Do you?

Those who lose their minds when provoked or attacked and turn an attacker into a victim while continuing to pound away at a now helpless person - taking out all their hate and frustrations on this person - really have to look in the mirror. They need to take a good look inside themselves. Is there really any peace in there? Unlikely.

It is true that we have what is commonly called an animal "survival instinct" and when threatened we may access what has been referred to as the "reptilian brain" where we can lose our human consciousness out of desperation and for survival.

Which is why when a person is physically attacked in any way and finds a way to turn the tables on their attacker, but loses control and takes it too far, should not, in my humble opinion, be held accountable in a court of law. Or, at the very least, this natural mechanism of survival should be strongly considered during the process, not side-stepped or left out of court and seen as a poor excuse because it is actually a valid reason.

How is it any different than "temporary insanity?"

I have one thing to say to the prosecutors, judges, and juries that disagree: have you ever experienced a situation like that for yourself first-hand? If not, then you have no right judging how someone else responds. You may very well respond the same way or worse if your life depended on it.

The only possibility of a fair trial is to have a jury full of people who have experienced a life-or-death attack for themselves. Only these people can relate. Only these people could evaluate based on personal experience, not theory. That would be a true jury of peers. One likely problem with that is most are probably dead.

But that's not how it works in court. Prosecutors are more concerned with winning than with the truth in many cases. They have a record to consider, just like they do in sports.

So if someone had an experience that helps them better relate to the defendant, most likely they would be excused from jury duty.

Am I wrong?

Our instinct is to survive, and once our ability to think is compromised due to fear and our inborn survival instincts, how can we be judged or held accountable?

Authorities will say it's a deterrent. That putting someone away is an example to others to maintain better control of themselves. But this misses the point. When you are in a life-or-death-situation, the average person is not able to weigh these legal consequences once their survival instincts take over. And it's not so easy to shut them down either. So the laws deter no one that gets to that point, and that should be recognized.

That's why there's the old saying in the martial arts:

"Better to be judged by twelve than carried by six."

That said, I am a strong advocate for proper training of the body *and the mind*. That is what martial arts training has always been for. You learn and practice to use the breath to control the mind. You meditate every day. Then, you'll be better equipped for stressful, in the moment, situational decisions.

That can save lives on both sides. And keep more unfortunate people out of prison as well (who successfully thwarted an attack but may have "lost it" or just went too far maybe even accidentally killing their assailant during the process).

What I have found in all my years and exposure to all kinds of people, both good and bad, is that a trained mind is a calm mind. A calm mind makes better decisions.

And, a calm mind finds having love, compassion, respect, and well wishes for everyone and everything... easy, regardless of what "they" do.

Winter Blues and the Power Inside

When the days are shorter, and it's dark or cold outside, it's very depressing for a lot of people. Is there anything we can do about that?

How is it any different than going through a "winter season" (difficult times) in your life?

It's really the same. You're not going to change the time of year. You're not going to change the sunset. And if you can recognize your inability to change the difficult situation you are facing, or something other people are doing that upsets you, then you know it is out of your power as well. No matter how upset you get over it, if there's nothing you can do there's nothing you can do.

Instead of dwelling on what you cannot change yet believe you can't stop thinking about, *focus on the things that make you feel better, and you will feel better.*

Do you have a pet? Do you have something in your life that makes you smile? Those who have a pet, like a dog, have a great experience to draw from. They go home, and their dog wants to jump out of their skin, they're so excited to see you, and their tail is wagging so hard it looks like it could come right off. All of you have to do is imagine that, and it makes you smile.

So you think about what makes you smile, whatever makes you feel good, in the moment that you don't feel so good, and watch how fast you can change your mind and your emotional state.

You have that power. *That is what you always have control over.*

But if you just want to focus on things like, "It's a lousy day..." then you're going to spiral down, feel worse. It's a focus, and it's a choice.

The first stage of meditation is your ability to concentrate. This is how you start to control your mind. You can decide to think of good things, or I should say: *one good thing*. Avoid thinking of more than one thing. As you attempt to focus on one thing at a time you may find your thoughts jumping all around. No worries. Just try to stay on the one thing you are choosing to focus on. And if you make that one thing that you focus on something that makes you smile...

It's difficult to feel bad when you're smiling. Then you'll realize how much control you really have over your experience in life. All you have to do is picture that thing that brings a smile to your face and bam, your face lights up. You forget what bothers you and better feelings will follow.

When "bad" things happen, and they happen to all of us, many will say, "But I can't stop thinking about it!"

This is your belief. You think you can't stop thinking about it. You absolutely can stop thinking about it by simply thinking of something else, something better, something that brings a smile to your face, instead.

However, chances are you'll keep going back to it because you want to change it. If you recognize you can't change it, it's a lot easier to let it go. You know how we argue with what is. We argue with it all the time, and that's why so many people live with so much stress.

Learn to accept and just let it go.

Think of the thing that makes you smile and go with it. This results in a much better life experience. Life is much more enjoyable that way.

Don't you agree?

If you want to feel bad, you can. If you want to feel good, you can. Just know it is your choice.

ADDENDUM

———◆———

If You Really Want To Experience A Powerful Life, Don't Leave This Out

This is a bonus section that I wanted to include because I find the physical self defense skills to be not only important but empowering.

Here, I discuss ways to end a fight without fighting, what it really means to be a martial artist (maybe not what you think!), and the ability to recognize potential life-threatening situations.

All components of martial arts must be considered if we truly want to enjoy "A Powerful Life." We should not deny the physical aspects of the training simply because we don't like fighting.

I don't like fighting either, but I love traditional martial arts. There is no conflict there, and the growth that can occur because of training with various partners, of all different shapes, sizes, and dispositions, in practice is something that transfers well into everyday life, where people don't think of you as a "partner."

I never want to hurt anyone. However, if someone attempts to bring physical harm to me, my wife, or my children I would not hesitate to do whatever is necessary. I will do anything in my power to be there for my family and loved-ones for years to come.

Any problem with that?

Well, with that said, I believe I have the responsibility to train myself to as high a level as I am able to reach so that in a moment of crisis, I will respond well and maintain as much control of the situation as possible. Hopefully, my skills allow me to get out of the situation without anyone being harmed. Including my assailant.

I often use this example with my students: training your physical skills to a high level is like having a gun in your back pocket. You know it's there if you need it, so your ability to keep calm and think clearly in the face of a threat is much easier.

You know what to do because you're prepared. You're not handcuffed by fear. You know your options and can now focus on diffusing the situation.

The first line of self defense is awareness. When you're aware of a potential danger, you at least have a chance to avoid it. If that fails, the next goal is to get out of the situation as quickly and safely as possible.

I do believe that a true martial artist takes responsibility for his or her own safety. We cannot always assume that we are safe, walking around with the proverbial bag over our heads, and that the authorities have us covered anytime and anywhere.

Not anymore.

How To Win A Fight Without Fighting

Proper training of the skills must include an intense focus on the body and or the partner (real or imagined - like shadow boxing). Any extraneous thoughts distract from the task at hand, and there was a time for martial artists when distraction could get you killed, just like any soldier in combat.

The physical side of martial arts training includes exercises for strength, endurance, flexibility, mobility, speed, power, balance and coordination among other things. This is the area that most people focus on when they look to "get in shape" by taking martial arts classes.

In the Chinese martial arts, good training includes the concept of *Yin* and *Yang* and the interaction of these opposing but complimentary aspects.

The Yang aspect is the physical side of training, and generally, *spends energy*. Think of the various strength and conditioning training that gets you breathing heavy and sweating a lot. It is also what builds you up and how your body responds according to the demands you're asking of it: to get stronger, more flexible, better mobility, balance, etc.

The Yin side, or "Internal" training aspect, is unfortunately, where most people neglect their practice. It is at least equal to if not more important than the physical side as it supports through better structural integration and protects the body from most detrimental effects from the physical side (such as repetitive use types of injuries).

The Yin aspect of the practice is also the key to reaching higher levels of focus, sensitivity, and awareness. Would those qualities be helpful to have more of in your life?

For a well-trained martial artist, the whole body must be used while executing a technique. Your ability to defend yourself cannot depend on you being bigger and stronger because that is rarely the case.

This kind of skill can only be achieved through inner calmness, deep relaxation (suppleness), structural integrity (posture), and the development of reflexive movements (to move without thinking).

Look especially to breathing, meditation and Qigong to develop the Yin side.

More Yin and Yang

How about avoiding a confrontation altogether and meeting aggression with a passive approach? Or staying calm in an argument?

Becoming angry will add fuel to the fire and escalate the problem. It doesn't matter if you think you are right, if you can let go of your ego and learn to remain calm and listen instead of forcing in your opinion or convincing others of your perspective, you will likely end up with a clearer understanding and a calmer situation.

Many times throughout my life, when someone learns what I do for a living they ask, "Have you ever had to use it?"

My response? "I use it every day."

Now I know they are only thinking about the kind of fighting they see in movies and on pay-per-view. Most seem to think that physical confrontation cannot be avoided in many cases.

Let me tell you, this is simply not accurate. Sure, there are exceptions, but it is not nearly as prevalent as many whose focus is on the physical side of self defense may have you think.

I've had my share of confrontational situations with some pretty bad people, the kind that fight at the drop of a hat. And yet, we did not fight.

Why?

Because I was not responding to their aggression in the way they expected.

I have found that when well trained in the physical techniques, it is akin to having a gun in the holster. You do not pull it out unless you intend to use it.

But if you do, someone is going to get hurt. And as I already stated, I have no desire to hurt anyone.

Isn't that precisely why we have thousands of nuclear weapons pointing at who our government sees as our enemies? We could blow up the whole planet many times over but then everyone loses. It is a deterrent in an effort to keep the peace.

When mentally and physically prepared for confrontation, you can more easily defuse the situation. It becomes easier to avoid a fight that, to many, may seem unavoidable.

That's because they let their ego and emotions get the best of them.

When you know what to do, it is far easier to remain calm and centered while facing a threat. You can maintain respect for their opinion and where they're coming from. You can allow them to keep their dignity and save face. You can consciously choose not to do anything that gets them further into their downward spiral into an animal mindset and the point of no return... when you're not in a panic yourself.

Then you can keep your focus on what the threat actually is. You can "watch your six" as well because you don't go into tunnel vision thinking the only threat is in front of you.

You can recognize and maintain safe distance and angles.

That's my only focus. I really don't listen to a word they're saying. Let them blow their top and say whatever they feel the need to say. Don't allow them to get in your head. Don't get offended or upset. Keep thinking and evaluating.

Your response, or lack thereof, can throw them off mentally to the point where they decide not to escalate further. And they calm down.

That's been my experience, and it would not have been possible without my training.

You see, I know that nobody really wins a fight.

They can say what they want to say and do just about anything short of physically crossing the line. I find it all irrelevant to whether we get into it or not... unless they cross the line physically where I have no choice unless I don't mind being injured or killed.

Short of that, I still have the choice not to fight.

This is the use of wisdom in self defense. In a fight that can be avoided, especially one that is fueled by ego, even if you win, you lose.

"Those who seek harmony know how to find it" - Chinese Proverb

The Reality of Self Defense

When people think about self defense, and training in the martial arts for that purpose, the focus is on learning to punch, block, lock, throw, and kick in some fashion. However, the mental/emotional side is far more important.

Chapter 33 of the Dao De Jing says it like this:

"Those who overcome others have strength; Those who overcome themselves are powerful."

Proper training in self defense reveals that awareness and avoidance can keep you out of harm's way and mindset can save you if some form of violence does find you.

Stranger Danger

Although many believe that it is just bad luck or "wrong place, wrong time," this is rarely the case. Victim selection is like a science for the criminal. There is nothing random about it.

In an old video by one self defense expert, Marc MacYoung, ("Safe in the Street," 1993) a study is mentioned where prison inmates were shown a short film of people walking in a crowded mall and were asked to choose who they believe would be a good victim candidate.

95% chose the same potential victims!

It's important to understand that prison is more of an inconvenience than a deterrent, with three square meals and free medical and dental. The criminal knows he won't be there long anyway. He is not afraid of prison - he is more concerned about being hurt or experiencing immediate pain.

He knows that if he is hurt, he can easily be preyed upon by others like him. His safety relies on *choosing the right victim.*

Criminals will try to remove your options - you either give in or get hurt. They don't want a fight. They want to get their way and be done with it.

The criminal will first check to see if you are safe to attack; and second, set up in a position that will limit your choices.

Becoming aware of your surroundings will very likely keep you out of harm's way at this stage of the game.

Take notice of people and places around you. Be aware of their position relative to yours. Is there someplace you can be cornered? Are there others around or are you alone? What is your gut feeling? Use common sense and change the scenario when necessary.

The Interview:

They'll read your body language from a distance. Being "trapped in your head" is perfect for them. You're already distracted.

Appearing timid, weak, or with general signs of low self-esteem and bingo, you're chosen for the next step; the interview.

Usually, the initial approach is a request for something. They don't care about the answer, they want to distract you, just long enough for their next move.

In the highly-recommended book, "The Gift of Fear," author Gavin De Becker runs off seven excellent "Survival Signals" for predicting ulterior motives and/or bad intent. The following is compiled from there with the author's words in quotes and italicized:

Forced Teaming - a *we're-in-the-same-boat* attitude is an effective way to establish premature trust. Using terms like: *"Both of us"; "We're some team"; "How are we going to handle this?"; "Now we've done it,"* etc., to put you on a fabricated common ground.

De Becker's suggested defense: *"I did not ask for your help, and I do not want it."* This may appear rude, but so what? If it is being used *"... by a stranger to a woman in a vulnerable situation (such as alone in a remote or unpopulated area), it is always inappropriate."*

Charm and Niceness – *"To charm is to compel, to control by allure or attraction."* Instead of "He's charming" as a description of a stranger's traits, see it as, "He's trying to charm me," as an action being carried out. Charm has motive. *De Becker says, "'He was so nice' is a comment I often hear from people describing the man who, moments or months after his niceness, attacked them."*

Too Many Details - *"When people are telling the truth, they don't feel doubted, so they don't feel the need for additional support in the form of details. When people lie,* *however, even if what they say sounds credible to you, **it doesn't sound credible to them**, so they keep talking."* This also works as a distraction. Always keep the context of the details in mind. Remember, this is a stranger who approached you.

I was once on one of my weekly trips to the Baltimore area for training when at a rest stop, and while walking back to my car with my hands full of food and drink, I was approached by a big burly individual. I immediately put my stuff down and looked around to see if there was anyone else approaching before putting all my attention on him.

He was going on and on about his truck and the troubles he was having as he approached. Clearly, he was telling me *too many details* to simply be legitimately asking for assistance. While facing him, maintaining a safe distance and gesturing with both hands up in front of me, I made it clear that any "help" he needed was inside the rest stop facility.

It became clear to him that I was on to whatever his plan was and he reluctantly moved on. I have no doubt what his intentions were. I trusted my gut instincts and you should too.

Typecasting - Being labeled in a slightly critical way in hope you'll feel compelled to prove the opinion is not accurate. *"You're probably too snobbish to talk to someone like me,"* and so you talk to him to prove you're not a snob. *"You don't look like someone who reads the newspaper,"* and you set out to show you are intelligent and well-informed.

You refuse someone's help and they say, *"There's such a thing as being too proud,"* so you accept their help to prove you're not.

No response is effective because it's the response itself that he's after. *"He doesn't believe what he said is true, he only believes it will work."*

Loan Sharking - When someone does something for you, it is difficult to not want to return the favor in some way, even if it is just being nice to them. This is known as the law of reciprocity. Getting him to leave you alone after he has helped you is much more difficult. Just remember, he approached you and you didn't ask for help.

The Unsolicited Promise - *"One of the most reliable signals because it is nearly always of questionable motive."* The reason a person would make an unsolicited promise is because he can see that you don't believe him.

Your body language is one of distrust. Now consider that if you didn't hear your intuition sooner, the one making promises is telling you that you don't trust him - like a second chance to read the signals of your intuition that you may have missed.

"Always, in every context, be suspicious of the unsolicited promise," says De Becker.

Keep yourself conscious of the situation by responding, at least to yourself, that "You're right, I don't trust you."

Discounting the Word, "No" – When a stranger ignores you and proceeds in spite of your refusals, De Becker says this is, *"Perhaps the most universally significant signal of all. The person who chooses not to hear 'no' is trying to control you, and once you give in, the stage is set for more effort to control.*

Defense: When someone ignores that word, ask yourself, 'Why is this person trying to control me? What does he want?'

If you can, get away. If you can't, this is a good time to raise your voice and be obnoxious. Look to attract attention (the one thing a criminal doesn't want). Say clearly, "I SAID NO!"

Intuition:

According to De Becker, if you recognize that you are being interviewed see it for what it is. This doesn't mean to walk around being paranoid as if every unexpected stranger you encounter is a criminal intent on harming you, *"...but it does mean that you react to the signals if and as they occur. Trust that what causes alarm probably should, because when it comes to danger, intuition is always right in at least two ways: 1) It is always in response to something; 2) It always has your best interest at heart."*

You Pass the Interview:

I should say failed, from your perspective. Well, at this point, I like the Golden Rules of self defense expert Tony Blauer: 1) Acceptance - the opposite of denial; 2) Get challenged - find your "ON" switch; and 3) Don't stop thinking - stay in the moment and focus on solutions, not imagined outcomes.

Know your A, B, C's:

Another helpful way to look at this and put it all together for easy recall is with our A, B, C's: By simply demonstrating *Awareness* we can greatly reduce our chances of getting "chosen" for a crime. Also, when aware we have a better shot at *Avoidance*. And, if you were unable to avoid the threat for whatever reason, *Acceptance* of the reality of the situation.

As discussed above on training the Yin side, a martial artist practices various *Breathing* techniques. The breath is the bridge between the mind and the body. In order to remain calm and centered while facing adversity or any difficult situation, lengthen and deepen your breathing (literally *deeper*, where your belly expands as you breathe in). Then, breathe out slower as well.

Quick shallow breaths, the norm for stressful situations, results in more stress and tension, generally making things worse with more difficulty thinking clearly or making decisions.

In order to keep thinking we must be able to calm down.

A shout of, "No!" is also a practical use of the breath. It can help you to *Break* the pattern of shock and fear, or the "deer in headlights" effect, getting you to do *something*.

Communicate clearly and *Confidently*. Mean what you say and don't allow your potential attacker to ignore your wish for them to leave you alone and move on. This communication includes how you move and appear to others (see below: "How

To Not Be Seen As A Good Victim"). So, walk confidently as well.

Decide what you must do, and do it. *Don't make things worse* by ignoring the signs that your intuition may be telling you, arguing, or fighting if you can avoid it. Again, **the goal in real self defense is to get out of the situation as quickly and as safely as possible, not to win a fight.**

Experience leads to confidence. The practice of martial arts, including preparing for possible scenarios, results in better decision-making skills if or when an emergency situation arises. Experience leads to recognition, which allows for a faster response and better chance to come out unscathed.

As you'll see again in the Situational Awareness chapter coming up, just as we prepare for the possibility of a fire with fire drills: if you are ever in a real life-threatening situation, would you rather have options that are known to be effective at your disposal or be totally guessing?

Mindset:
The right mindset has saved many lives. Little 80-pound Kate O'Leary, the wife of an over twenty-year student, James O'Leary, told me a story of how she was once approached for money by a group of teenagers. Let's just say she scared the snot out of them and they ran off with nothing!

How To Not Be Seen As A Good Victim
If you've ever had the opportunity to watch how the various styles of martial artists from around the world move, you may have noticed the smooth, fluid and circular emphasis of the Chinese martial arts in particular. It is noticeably different than the harder styles of the East such as Karate or Tae Kwon Do. The movements display more lightness and grace.

Well, according to a study by Betty Grayson and Morris I. Stein published way back in 1981 (and referenced many times since) "Attracting Assault: Victims' Nonverbal Cues," the very traits developed by practitioners of Kung Fu make them inherently less likely to ever have to defend themselves!

Let me explain: Grayson and Stein made videotapes of random people walking on the street in New York City, in an area with one of the highest assault rates, and then showed the recordings to a group of prison inmates. These inmates were all "convicted of assaultive crimes ranging from murder to simple assault on victims unknown to them."

The inmates then rated the "assault potential" of the people in the recordings. According to the results of the study, "… mean differences between victims and non-victims in rated assault potential were rather large."

You'd think that the smallest women would be selected as victims and the larger men would be categorized as "non-victims," but that wasn't the case. In fact, quite the opposite occurred in some cases. How could this be?

Well, one of the more obvious answers to that question was already discussed above: looking like you're aware and not distracted. Also, appearing purposeful and confident. However, the study found something very different when the people selected were studied with a fine-toothed comb.

So, what were the main criteria for selection realized through analysis? *How they moved!*

Specifically, the study found that, "… stride length, type of weight shift, type of walk, body movement, and feet" were the main factors giving off "easy target" signals to the criminals.

According to a Psychology Today article that referenced this study (January 1, 2009, "Marked For Mayhem" by Chuck Hustmyre and Jay Dixit), *"The researchers realized the criminals were assessing the ease with which they could overpower the targets based on several nonverbal signals - posture, body language, pace of walking, length of stride, and awareness of environment. Neither criminals nor victims were consciously aware of these cues. They are what psychologists call 'precipitators,' personal attributes that increase a person's likelihood of being criminally victimized."*

The authors go on to say, *"The researchers analyzed the body language of the people on the tape, and identified several aspects of demeanor that marked potential victims as good targets. One of the main precipitators is a walking style that lacks 'interactional synchrony' and 'wholeness.' Perpetrators notice a person whose walk lacks organized movement and flowing motion. Criminals view such people as less self-confident - perhaps because their walk suggests they are less athletic and fit - and are much more likely to exploit them."*

What this means for the practitioner of a style of traditional Kung Fu, especially the art of Ba Gua Zhang, an art known for its footwork and smooth mobility, is that the training itself greatly reduces ever having to use it in a physical confrontation. You are simply far more likely to be left alone by the criminal intent on assault.

Of course, there are many athletic pursuits that can result in "moving better," but add to that the calmer, more peaceful, and respectful approach of a traditionally trained martial artist, as discussed above, and you can virtually eliminate conflict in your life... especially the physical kind.

So, what does it mean to be a martial artist?

What It Means To Be
A Martial Artist

I hope at this point I have made it clear that martial arts are not all about fighting and violence. Quite the opposite actually.

However, if you're training in the martial arts and not learning how to defend yourself, can you still consider yourself a martial artist?

Or, is it a term reserved only for Bruce Lee, Chuck Norris, or the Jason Bourne-like characters we see in the movies?

Maybe you think it's just the pay-per-view MMA fighters?

Are students seeing something that is beyond their ability to reach? Is it an ideal, unrealistic in their lives?

If so, this is a good reason why most just dabble in the martial arts, never really getting out of it what they had hoped for. They have a dream or visions of grandeur thinking, "It would be cool if...", but cannot see it as a reality in the end. It remains nothing but a fantasy for those who give up too soon.

The truth is, *anyone* who sets their mind to it, has some patience and perseveres, can get everything martial arts training has the potential to provide, which is usually far more than was ever expected.

The Chinese Character That Translates to "Martial"

The Chinese character that was translated to the word "martial" is *wu* (武). And if we break down the character (*ge*, 戈, "spear" + *zhi*, 止, "stop") it literally means, "to stop the use of weapons," "to end the violence," or "to stop the fighting."

It is for this primary reason that we have the mightiest and most advanced military on the planet: to end conflict so we can enjoy peace.

A martial artist, *whose main goal is peace*, develops the expertise, the skills, the techniques, and all the tools necessary *to end conflict.*

We must be careful when we try to stretch out or too loosely interpret the meaning of martial arts and what it means to be a martial artist.

We cannot leave out the physical aspect.

To be truly prepared to end the conflict it means that if it escalates to that point you are still prepared.

Can You Say You're a Martial Artist if You're Not Sparring?

I'm not talking about sparring in a competitive way, where one wins, and the other loses. Not with a focus on tournaments and trophies, where one plans and prepares for a match.

I mean sparring in a way where you practice the physical skills that can help you stop the fight. Because that's the goal: not to win, not for tournaments, not for trophies, not to beat people up, not to compete but *to end the conflict* and ultimately live in peace.

What's the difference between real self defense and competitive fighting or combat sports?

In a real self defense situation, there is no scheduled encounter. There is surprise and many times shock. And there are no rules.

Fighting competitions and combat sports like MMA have nothing to do with whether one is a martial artist - or isn't. We just must see it for what it is: a competitive *sport.*

How's this for a definition of a martial artist:

One who studies, practices, develops, and creatively expresses the tools, techniques, and skills to face adversity and end conflict - from the inner battle up to and including a physical confrontation.

We Don't All Have To Be Green Berets

There are many levels of preparedness. The more prepared you are, the more likely it is that you can decide not to turn to violence and avoid or end conflict.

There are the specialists, such as the Green Berets or Special Forces, who are trained to face the most dangerous life-threatening situations.

And then there is the mother who maintains peace in the home by mediating and softening the atmosphere when there is conflict within the family. This mother has highly developed *people skills,* also known as diplomacy.

Yes, people skills are another significant tool in the martial artist's arsenal. It is people skills that allow us to end conflict before it escalates.

An Old Master Of Karate Told Me...

In Okinawan Karate, they have titles beyond the first three Dan of black belt.

At the 4th to 6th Dan, the title is *Renshi.*

At the 7th and 8th Dan, the title is *Kyoshi.*

And at the 9th and 10th Dan, the highest levels, the title is *Hanshi.*

Why the titles, and what do they say about the meaning of being a martial artist?

Renshi means, "polished." *Kyoshi* means, "more polished." And *Hanshi*, the highest level? Simply "even more polished."

Polished what?

Character.

The true martial artist is always making efforts to better himself - striving for perfection - to be impeccable in all that he does.

She knows that before she can control anything, self-control must come first. If we are conflicted within, how can we seriously expect to end conflict anywhere else?

How Our Motto Results In Less Conflict:

Wisdom: Accumulated knowledge and experience to consciously apply the tools, techniques, and skills to end conflict - within and without; think before you act. The wise person makes better decisions.

Benevolence: Thinking of others; concern for others; respect. If you show others respect, you'll have less conflict. No one is better or more important than anyone else.

Sincerity: Truthful and honest with yourself and others - especially about your efforts or lack thereof. Living in accordance with who you really are results in less *inner* conflict.

Bravery: There is no bravery without fear. When uncomfortable, you do it anyway. Facing fear leads to confidence. A confident person has nothing to prove so allows others to be who they are and have their own perspectives and opinions. Therefore, there is more acceptance and less conflict.

The Confidence Of Knowing What To Do

Again, the gun in the back pocket gives more confidence. When you really know you are prepared to handle the worst-case scenario - including escalation to a physical confrontation - you can better focus on *diffusion*.

You can have thoughts such as, "How can I throw water on this fire?" rather than being full of fear of where it may be going - and frozen, unable to do anything about the situation -- or having an emotional knee-jerk reaction that can easily make things worse.

Confidence allows for calmness and calmness allows for clarity. You can keep thinking - which is essential in life-threatening situations.

But this calm and centered demeanor is also contagious.

If you can stay calm while the other is losing it in anger, they are very likely to pick up on your lack of fear or emotional response and either lose confidence themselves (as they begin to realize you're not an easy victim) or simply calm down as a result - all depending on the situation (criminal or domestic).

What is your attitude? Is it bringing water or more fire to the situation?

The Immovable Mind

Musashi, the famous Samurai, spoke of this concept of the "rock body" - or "immovable mind" of the martial artist - indifferent to the goings on around him. Regardless of the circumstances, mentally and emotionally, he is the same. Whether in a life or death situation or having tea with a friend, he is unattached and unaffected.

In the Chinese "Five Elements," the rock is Metal.

Metal creates Water. Water controls Fire.

Your calmness or immovable mind and indifference toward whether the situation escalates or resolves *becomes the water that can put out the fire of aggression.*

This is another important application of Yin and Yang when it comes to self defense: *"Kan and Li"* (representing two of the "Eight Trigrams," or *Ba Gua*, "Water" and "Fire," respectively). Fire, brings the fight. This is the aggressor.

Water, on the other hand, waits for the fight to come to them; it's having the attitude of "You'll have to bring it to me." If no one is the aggressor, there is no fight.

The martial artist does not want to fight. Therefore, he or she studies and develops the skills so that he or she does not have to. *The highest level of fighting is not to fight.*

Therefore, it's always better to be like Water, right?

Not necessarily. Sometimes Fire is necessary. If you are close enough to the doorway where an armed lunatic (active shooter) enters, as it went down in the Orlando night club, June 12, 2016, and you are aware (as you should always be paying attention to your surroundings, especially in this day and age) the best course of action is to quickly attack this person and attempt to disable him. Move off the line from the barrel of the gun, grab hold of his head with both hands, and throw your thumbs into their eyes! Do whatever it takes! (Gory, I know, but that's bravery, by the way.)

In this example, Water, or being passive and waiting, will get you killed.

Of course, if you don't happen to be close enough, then quickly find cover and get away as quickly as possible.

So When Are You a Martial Artist?

Is it only when you have mastered all of the above and more, skillfully and reflexively responding most appropriately in any given situation?

Remember this: mastery is a process.

Let's say, at the very least, you are a martial artist if you are *continually working toward* acquiring and accumulating the knowledge and experience necessary to end conflict within yourself, in your life and ultimately the world, including the tools, techniques, and skills to deal with people on all levels.

From raising happy, healthy, confident children...

to personal or work-related relationships...

to facing personal fears and overcoming limiting beliefs...

to that worst-case scenario wrong place wrong time physical encounter with the crack-addicted criminal where you are nothing more to him than a way to get his next hit...

the martial artist is always learning, training, and preparing... so he or she can live the most fulfilling, peaceful, and awakened life.

So... *are you a martial artist?*

Next, a further shift into personal safety: Should a martial artist who just wants to live a happier, healthier life be concerning themselves with terrorist and terrorist-like events that have become a far too frequent occurrence throughout the world?

Turn the page to see what maybe hasn't occurred to you about it...

Keeping Safe With
Situational Awareness

The title of this book, "It's A Powerful Life" is meant to suggest that it is about self-empowerment. A powerful life, to me, is one where I am happy, healthy, strong and confident. It also suggests a sense of control and that I am also free to choose what I do with my life.

Fear runs many people's lives. There's fear of failure, fear of not being accepted, fear of new things, and of course, fear of the dangerous world we live in.

How can you expect to live "a powerful life" if you're run by fear? How can you consider yourself free if you're decisions come from a lack of confidence or courage?

We fear most what we know the least about. Fear has also been made into an acronym: False Evidence Appearing Real. In other words, our imagination runs wild and what we think we know about something trumps the truth about that thing.

Knowledge is power. Knowledge coupled with experience brings wisdom and confidence. From there, courage can grow and crush this kind of fear.

As a lifetime martial artist, I believe strongly in preparing for "what if" scenarios. If I learn more about what I fear I can take away any power that thing has over me and how I live my life. By educating myself in the kinds of things that can threaten my health, happiness or wellbeing, I am empowered.

Preparation gives you viable options in an emergency or life-threatening situation when there may be no time at all to think and make a decision. Surprise is a cousin to fear. Preparation reduces the chance of being surprised.

A wise person prepares by considering the possibilities that may arise. To me, that too is empowering.

When I share what I have discovered so that others are empowered, I feel like I have done my part to help improve, and maybe even save, the lives of others as well.

That's What This Chapter is About...

This chapter may not seem to fit into a "self-help" sort of book, but it was inspired by events that occurred at the Pulse nightclub in Orlando, Florida in the early morning hours of Sunday, June 12, 2016, near closing time.

When I came into our evening classes the Monday after, I had a little something to say about it in each class. I believe it is important to address these unexpected, horrific events that plague our society.

On the one hand, we can become depressed, demoralized, defeated, and live in fear, avoiding to live our lives to the fullest. On the other hand, we can look as a martial artist should and ask, "What can I do about it?"

Any situation that you face, any tough challenge you have in life, whatever problems you have, the focus shouldn't be so much on the problem. It should be on the solution.

What can I do in this situation? And when your life falls apart, rugs pulled out from you, the mind must focus on, "What can I do?" rather than focusing on how bad it is and "Whoa is me."

Also, simply acknowledging the suffering of others so far away, having compassion, shedding a few tears and feeling empathy while remaining in denial that it can or will happen to you, no matter how statistically impossible it may seem, may be very naive as these events are increasing in frequency.

Let me ask one question: Would you rather be prepared and know what to do and have it never happen, or be in the middle of the next night club (or wherever) attack and not have a clue?

We all become far more aware of these things when it's fresh in our minds after an attack. However, we are soon lulled right back into oblivion and the busy-ness of our lives.

No Down Time

I regularly remind students that there is no downtime. But let's get realistic - we have down time. It's just that I encourage the diligent approach to always be aware - of your actions, reactions, decisions, posture, and of course your surroundings.

That's why this event hit me harder than even the school shootings where small children lost their lives. Not because one is any worse than the other (actually the slaughter of children should make anyone sick to their stomachs) but because children aren't able or expected to protect themselves. They need our protection.

However, in the Orlando nightclub, they were adults. Should adults be putting their full-time protection in the hands of others? As a martial artist, I have to say no. We are each responsible for our own safety first.

So, here they are, out having some fun, fully believing they were perfectly safe. It could be any one of us. Anyone reading this has these fun times (hopefully!) because we must have what most would consider "downtime" in life.

But that's what hit me so hard. As an instructor who cares deeply for his students, and that as martial artists in training, what can I do so it doesn't happen to one of them, or me? Have I done all I can? Can I, should I do better?

Expanding Experience

Every year, we have a two-and-a-half day retreat out in nature. Since the art we practice is based on natural laws, experiencing more of what nature has to offer, first-hand, can have a profound effect on our practice.

We've done all sorts of things from Native American awareness drills to experiencing other related Chinese martial arts such as Tai Ji Quan or Xing Yi Quan.

We've also done knife defenses, gun disarms, how to deal with a club or pipe being swung at you, etc. It's been a number of years, and we like to mix it up.

Well, based on feedback, by far this past year's favorite part was when we worked with realistic metal and weight equivalent Airsoft guns for the disarms and had a whole discussion on this situational awareness and active shooter problem.

My original plan was to do a mock "active shooter" event using one of these guns which have a realistic blowback that can sound like real live rounds going off. This was going to allow people to safely experience first-hand how they might respond when they don't expect it. I was going for a dose of reality so that they could become more prepared if it ever happened where they were for real.

Unfortunately, when I let the people who were in charge of the retreat facilities know so that they wouldn't freak out themselves, they shut it down. They didn't want anything to do with it, not even the perfectly safe sound of gun shots by gas blowback. I wasn't even going to shoot blanks here, just air (or gas actually). Ironically, there was a nearby neighbor who was clearly shooting at something on and off.

I get it. I respected their concerns and decision. However, to me, this was like sticking your head in the sand and either ignoring the very real threat we all face today or simply being naive enough to think "it won't happen to me."

You'd think they'd be curious and interested to see it for themselves, but no. Instead, it was a lost opportunity for people to learn something that could save their life one day.

All I want is to know as a martial arts instructor is that I've provided every chance for my students to be mentally and emotionally as well as physically prepared for the worst-case scenarios.

It is far better to be over prepared and never need to use it rather than have to actually face a totally unexpected life-or-death situation and become the deer in headlights having no idea whatsoever.

Which would you rather be?

When you've prepared for the worst, you have options. Why else would we have fire drills? However, a fire is just one possible emergency situation. Why not prepare for other possibilities as well?

Shift of Focus

If you focus on what happened, you're more likely to get broken down. You spend your time and energy (and conversations) on "What's this world coming to?" and the terrorists, and every other thing that's related. It spirals out of control without much going toward a solution other than killing all the terrorists (never happen) and eliminating guns (to be addressed below).

What we need to ask is, "What can I do to possibly prepare for the next one?" Because you never know if you just happen to be there. And there will be a next one. Why? Because we never get to the root of the problem.

Guns Don't Kill People. People Kill People.

I'm not trying to be political here, I just want to say that it's not the guns. And yes, I'd really prefer to have one and never need it than to not have one if anyone ever points one in my face (or starts shooting anywhere near me).

Until we get to the bottom of why people kill people, it will not stop, and we each have the God-given right to be able to protect ourselves.

The real question is: why is it increasing? One answer that I think is appropriate is that people are frustrated. The average person is working too much, not sleeping enough, eating things that do not nourish the body or the brain, and feels like they are barely keeping up or just keep going backward, all while looking for someone to blame for why their life is the way it is.

Here's a possibility:

According to the Citizens Commission on Human Rights, *"At least 35 school shootings and/or school-related acts of violence have been committed by those taking or withdrawing from psychiatric drugs resulting in 169 wounded and 79 killed (in other school shootings, information about their drug use was never made public-neither confirming or refuting if they were under the influence of prescribed drugs). The most important fact about this list, is that these are only cases where the information about their psychiatric drug use was made public."* (see: https://www.cchrint.org/school-shooters/)

But I digress.

If you still think it's the guns, well, in China private citizens are not allowed to possess firearms. Yet...

"33 Dead, 130 Injured in China Knife-Wielding Spree"

On the evening of March 1, 2014, at least 29 were killed and 130 were wounded at a train station in China. According to CNN: *"... 10 men armed with long knives stormed the station in the southwest Chinese city of Kunming, the state news agency Xinhua reported."*

"Members of a separatist group from Xinjiang, in northwest China, are believed to have carried out the assault, authorities said. The report referred to them as "terrorists."

"The killing spree came out of nowhere."

One witness stated, *"We saw two people carrying big cleavers hacking whoever is in the way."*

NBC News reported: *"Yunnan province Vice Gov. Gao Feng held an emergency meeting at No. 1 People's Hospital, where the injured are being rushed, and said hospitals have received 162 people."* Their updated headline stated, *"33 Dead, 130 Injured in China Knife-Wielding Spree"*

Not a gun in sight.

Here's an article reporting:

"Nine suspects are being pursued after they launched a coordinated knife attack and killed 50 workers at a northwestern Chinese coal mine, reports Radio Free Asia.

The incident occurred on September 18 in the Xinjiang Uyghur Autonomous Region. The attackers are alleged to be Uyghur separatists.

After overtaking security guards, the attackers killed the workers while they were asleep in bunkhouses at the Sogan colliery in Aksu. Another 50 workers were injured."

Some more updated details:

"An area double the size of Manhattan has been cordoned off as authorities pursue suspects following a coordinated knife attack that killed 60 workers at a northwestern Chinese coal mine, reports the FT." (Financial Times).

Then there are also far too many non-gun related school attacks as well:

"A man wielding a knife attacked students Friday at a school in central China, leaving 22 children and one adult injured, according to state-run media reports."

I know, with this one you're probably thinking "at least they weren't killed!"

Unfortunately, there are plenty more, as the same CBS News article continues:

"The attack marks the latest in a series of violent assaults at elementary schools in China. In 2010, a total of 18 children were killed in four separate attacks. On March 23 of that year, Zheng Minsheng attacked children at an elementary school in Fujian Province, killing eight.

One month later, just a few hours after Zheng Minsheng was executed for his crime, another man, Chen Kanbing wounded 16 students and a teacher in a knife attack at another primary school in Fujian. The following month, on May 12, a man named Wu Huangming killed seven children and two adults with a meat cleaver at a kindergarten in Shaanxi Province. That attack was followed by an August 4 assault by Fang Jiantang, who killed three children and one teacher with a knife at a kindergarten in Shandong Province.

In 2011, a young girl and three adults were killed with an axe at an elementary school in Henan Province by a 30-year-old man named Wang Hongbin, and eight children were hurt in Shanghai after an employee at a child care center attacked them with a box cutter."

So there are plenty of examples of disenchanted people still killing where guns are illegal for citizens to own.

In Seconds, I Was Able to Take Out 10 Myself...

Just to make a point at a social gathering where there was some anti-gun sentiment, armed with a plastic knife I was able to easily (pretend) to take out about 10 people in seconds, as I quickly moved around the room pretending to be "cutting their throats." I showed them how fast you can be killed with a knife. (Relax, not only was it plastic, I used the dull side.)

You press in on the neck and cut the carotid artery or right through and into the trachea and that's all she wrote. There's no time to save you. One, two, three, four, five... I just went from one to the other, weaving in and out between them (good ol' Ba Gua footwork!).

Then I said, "And you all think it's the guns."

It Doesn't Even Have to Be A Knife...

When someone knows what they're doing and are determined to do harm, they can kill with a pen, among other things that can be brought through airport security.

No guns were needed on 9/11. Apparently, box cutters were used in flight to take control of the planes.

In 2013, two homemade pressure cooker bombs were used in the Boston Marathon bombings. The bombers filled them with nails, ball bearings, and black powder.

Trucks Too...

Then there is the July 15, 2016, Bastille Day truck attack in Nice, France. According to CNN:

"Scores of people were killed Thursday night when a large truck plowed through a Bastille Day crowd in Nice, France, in what President Francois Hollande called a terror attack.

The death toll grew through the night, with Hollande saying 77 people died. Interior Minister Bernard Cazeneuve said 80 people were killed.

The driver first shot a gun into the crowd before driving two kilometers along the Promenade des Anglais, the main street in Nice, mowing down people who had gathered to watch fireworks, regional President Christian Estrosi told CNN affiliate BFM-TV."

Even while editing this book another attack occurred. Here is the CNN headline on December 19, 2016:

"Berlin Christmas market: 12 dead, 48 hospitalized in truck crash"

Darran Simon, Ralph Ellis and Frederik Pleitgen of CNN report: *"A tractor trailer barreled into a crowded Christmas market in Berlin on Monday night, killing 12 people and injuring 48 others. Witnesses said shoppers screamed and dropped packages and glasses of mulled wine as the truck plowed into the market.*

Officials are investigating the crash as an act of terrorism, according to a German intelligence official familiar with the matter."

Again, this isn't meant to be political. It's meant to be about what's going on in people's heads. Can we keep the guns away from the ones who are crazy? I'm sure they're working on it. I'm sure much smarter people than me are working on it.

However, it's not as simple as "stop the guns" because unfortunately, the bad people will have them and the good people won't. It's no different than a lock. Locks are for honest people.

Those who want to steal something break through locks, so it's not that. There is a psychological aspect.

Remember, the real meaning of "Kung Fu" (achievement through consistent effort over time) and the Chinese word for "martial," *Wu*, translates literally as *"stop the violence."*

Martial arts are the skills or the study of how to stop the violence. And it starts from within.

Situational Awareness

I hope I made my point. Guns don't kill people, people kill people. Your only defense is awareness, or more specifically, "Situational Awareness."

This is the kind of awareness the Secret Service must have to protect the President. The same for a deployed soldier in the field.

And that's what a trained martial artist carries into his or her day-to-day life. You cannot expect the authorities to protect you anytime, anywhere. That is your responsibility, like it or not.

What can we do? From the youth program up, I teach that the number one line of self defense is *awareness*. It's not about punching and kicking. Most people think self defense is fighting. Self defense is awareness. You will be far safer just by being aware of your surroundings.

So it's one thing for people to talk about being in the moment, and that's very helpful, but am I, in the moment, caught up in what I'm doing or am I in the moment aware of all that's going on around me? These are two different things. It depends on the environment.

There is an excellent book that I highly recommend, entitled, *Left of Bang,* by Patrick Van Home. The whole concept is this: "Right of bang" is after the attack, responding to it. This is where we're focused when we think that we need to be able to fight to defend ourselves. In many cases, it's already too late.

"Left of bang," on the other hand, means *before the attack.* What happens before the attack? What should we all be looking for?

That is the most valuable and practical information for self defense, or simply keeping yourself and your loved ones safe.

It started out as a course for Marines, but it has found its way into the private sector, and anyone willing can study in depth at the author's website: www.cp-journal.com. I've taken all levels and found them excellent.

Now, even if you just read the book, you'll be head and shoulders above most people (who generally have their head in the sand about these things).

It's one thing to be aware or mindful as diligently as possible and at all times. It's quite another to know what it is you should be looking for. You have to know what to do with the information you take in. And that's where the ball can be dropped.

That's why I decided to add this section and take advantage of this opportunity with you. As a martial arts instructor, I believe it's my responsibility, at the very least, to point you in the right direction, to help you start to realize what is happening around you and what to do with that information based on those surroundings, at the most basic level. You have other resources to take it further if you so choose.

OODA

U.S. Air Force fighter pilot and Pentagon consultant, Colonel John Boyd, came up with, "OODA," the acronym for, "Observe, Orient, Decide, and Act."

There are many accounts of people who were, for example, in 9/11 when the World Trade Center came down or various other tragedies. The people who survived are the ones who responded quickly. Those who respond to the warning, "There's an emergency! There's a fire! Get out of the building!" by going to collect their personal items... They don't make it out. Those who just get the message and go, they make it. Those are the ones telling the story. How did you get out? "Well, as soon as I heard, I went to the exit." "I went to the elevator." "I went to the stairwell right away, no hesitation." Those who hesitated weren't able to tell their stories.

Unfortunately, that's what those who were interviewed saw. They saw some people go back to get something important, "I gotta go get my bag. I gotta go get..." There is nothing important enough (phone, notes, files, keepsake, etc.) to lose your life over.

One survivor of the World Trade Center I met recently told me that when the first tower was hit, he left everything and went directly to the exit. And that's why he was able to tell me that in person sixteen years later.

The problem is, you have no idea how much time you have.

Somebody warns you. Think about all the steps that occurred and time that passed for that person to get the message to you. Already so much time was lost.

As soon as you observe the situation, you have to orient yourself for what to do.

The Cooper Color Code System

Then there is Lieutenant Colonel Jeff Cooper, who came up with a color code system. This is really effective, and everyone from the military to law enforcement to self defense experts have been incorporating this system into their instruction. Many, including the U.S. government, have altered and or expanded upon Cooper's original ideas, which I won't do here (if I can help it).

According to Cooper, "As I have long taught, you are not in any color state because of the specific amount of danger you may be in, but rather in a mental state which enables you to take a difficult psychological step."

The original Cooper Color Code System is: White, Yellow, Orange, and Red.

In the most abbreviated description I could find, in Vol. 13, No. 7 of "Jeff Cooper's Commentaries" (July 2005), Cooper wrote:

*"In **White,** you are unprepared and unready to take lethal action. If you are attacked in White, you will probably die unless your adversary is totally inept.*

In **Yellow,** *you bring yourself to the understanding that your life may be in danger and that you may have to do something about it.*

In **Orange,** *you have determined upon a specific adversary and are prepared to take action which may result in his death, but you are not in a lethal mode.*

In **Red,** *you are in a lethal mode and will shoot if circumstances warrant."*

Let me elaborate just a bit:

Condition White is basically when you walk around with a paper bag over your head, completely unaware of what's going on around you. You know, walking around with headphones on or texting or being engaged with anything other than what you're doing while out in public. You're in your own world basically.

You should never ever be in public wearing headphones and listening to music or whatever, or head down looking at your phone and texting. You are an opportunity for the criminal and or an accident waiting to happen.

Just last night, I was in Manhattan. Although it was dark out (and crowded as usual), there were numerous people walking around looking at their phones and texting. This was both on the sidewalk *and while crossing the street!*

Are you kidding me??

I discussed this in the chapter on perspective, but there it had more to do with how you feel about what others do such as who is at fault. Here the focus is on your safety. So let me repeat here, it doesn't matter whose fault it is legally. If you are walking across a crosswalk with your head down because you have the right of way and get hit by a car, you may be right, but you may also be killed!

When the Orlando nightclub shooting occurred, there was one video I saw that was most telling. You may have seen the girl with the glasses. She was talking to someone (on Facetime, I figure), so it's a video of her talking to somebody. When the gunshots go off in the background... *pop, pop, pop, pop...,* you can see her reaction. All she did was make an annoyed look (apparently because it was interrupting her conversation) and then kept on talking. She didn't respond with any sort of concern like, "What was that?!?", flinching or ducking her head down. She didn't turn to look and see what it was exactly. She just continued about her business.

Now, even if firecrackers went off, wouldn't you instantly turn and maybe raise your hands and or duck your head? She just looked annoyed as if thinking there is just someone being immature and making it difficult for her conversation. It didn't occur to her in the least that she was in grave danger. She was in full Condition White.

As far as I know, she didn't make it. Maybe if she did look to see what was actually happening, she would have had the time to run and get out alive. Unfortunately, for most people, the reality of what's happening doesn't set in.

That's why we all need to learn: *observe... orient...*

So, Condition White is completely unaware. You don't even observe. But if you do observe imminent danger, do you freeze? You know, the deer in headlights. You have to orient yourself to "What does this mean?" so you can get out of the situation as quickly as possible if you have a chance.

Yellow is where we need to be. Yellow is relaxed and alert, or simply relaxed alertness.

There have been many times when I've spoken to people or written about awareness and I explain how I'll walk out my door and take notice of things such as the two squirrels over there rustling in the leaves or the birds in the trees and how they're talking to each other, and the blue car going by... and I just take it all in. Why? Because I practice doing that.

Then someone may ask, "Shifu, isn't that stressful? Isn't that like being paranoid?"

Not at all. That's why I said, what does it mean to *be in the moment?*

Every single time I get on my motorcycle, every single time I get in the car, I am always working on seeing both sides of the street and even both rearview mirrors (for what's behind - not easy) with my peripheral vision. I keep my field of vision as big as I can. All the time I'm taking in all I can see. Driving down the highway I may see the American flag waving, and I see a car pull out, and I always work on picking things up before they happen (like brake lights going off a few cars ahead instead of just the one in front of me).

I used to joke that you can see the squirrel thinking about crossing the road instead of suddenly being in front of you and "Oh, my God!" As you slam on the breaks. You really can see them think about it. I'm joking, but I'm not joking. It really happens just like that.

Try it for yourself. You'll see you can catch them with your peripheral vision.

However, when you're in your own world, into your music and tunnel vision, you don't see anywhere near as much, and things can surprise you. You're much easier to be caught off guard.

So it's an on-going practice - relaxed and alert. There is no difference between Condition White and Condition Yellow as far as your heart rate. That's what's interesting. You're just as relaxed, it's just that White is in your own world and Yellow is what's going on in the environment around you. You're not just lost in your head.

How about Condition Orange? This is where you lock on to something specific as a possible threat. Your attention is focused on what you've observed, without losing track of the rest of the environment (someone distracting you from the front so their partner can attack from behind, for example). This is where you really want to know your options and only those who've prepared ahead of time will be able to respond the quickest (where every second counts and life or death can be determined).

Red is simply following through according to what you have observed and once you have oriented yourself. It's the willingness to do what you must, which may include taking a life, in order to assure your safety or the safety of someone you are protecting.

Here are a few examples that hopefully help to illustrate the difference between Condition Orange and Condition Red (or a return to Condition Yellow):

Orange: You see a car is headed right for you... Red: jump out of the way!

Orange: You smell smoke... realize your whole house is on fire... Red: get out!

Orange: Sounds like gun shots... realize it's just firecrackers... back to Condition Yellow

Orange: Sounds like gun shots... sudden chaos, people dropping, screaming, running... Red: Run - Hide - Fight!

Run - Hide - Fight!

According to the Department of Homeland Security, this is where you either run, hide, or fight. You know something is happening, and you must respond.

Through my research, I've discovered that the best thing to tell your children in an active shooter situation is not to hide and wait for help. That's what they did in Sandy Hook, Columbine, and Virginia Tech. The victims were sitting ducks, having made it very easy for their killers.

Unfortunately, this is how most school systems are trained to respond. By the time help arrives it can be too late for too many. It usually is in those situations.

Instead, I tell my kids to get out and run as fast as they can away from the school. Break a window if they have to and get out.

I realize that's the last thing the school Board wants to hear because they are responsible for what happens to the kids in school. But there are times and situations where they are not able to protect those children. I'd rather my children break the rules and survive rather than follow the rules and become a statistic.

Personal safety is an attitude and approach to how you do things. Do you regularly put yourself in harm's way? In his book, "Principles of Personal Defense," Jeff Cooper says, *"No sensible person ever opens the door of his house without knowing who is knocking."*

Seems like common sense, but many people have gotten themselves raped or murdered by doing just that. They *thought* they were safe because they were home. They were wrong.

Complacency is Pervasive

I recently had to pick up our daughter at school. She had a fever and the school wanted her picked up early. Usually, it's my wife who they see, however, on this day she was too far away and couldn't make it.

The school has the door locked, and you have to ring the bell for them to let you in. So I rang, and they buzzed to unlock the door.

See a problem with that yet? I took notice.

Strike one.

Then, I walked in, and a little unsure of where I had to go, wandered around just a bit. No one noticed.

Strike two.

I find the office and ask for my daughter by name. I'm pointed towards the nurse's office, and there I see her. I'm then told about her condition, and that she has to stay home the next day.

"Okay," I respond.

Then, as we're about to leave, the school nurse asks me for identification. Here comes strike three.

I asked the woman who buzzed me in if she knew who I was before letting me in. She said, "No."

And now they want identification? "Too late," I said.

Strike three.

I let them know what just happened. Their response? "We wouldn't have let you take her." Really? Like I said, too late. They need to know who it is they're letting in. Otherwise, what is the point of locking the door?

If I was one of those lunatics like the one who shot up the kids in Sandy Hook, it was too late. I was in, and I could have easily gone right down the hall and shot up as many children and adults as I encountered in the hallways and in the classrooms.

By the time help arrived, the damage would have been done. And that's why these attacks will continue - complacency. We make it so easy for them. I refuse to live that way, (oblivious to these possibilities) and I teach my children the best I can: If anything like that ever happens, get out and run as far away from that school as you can. Like I said, break a window to get out if you have to.

By the way, I must add that at Sandy Hook Elementary, they had the same security system in place. The shooter simply shot out the glass next to the locked door and proceeded to enter.

We must do better. At the very least, every school should be trained for these possible situations, regardless of how remote it may seem. How about installing a camera at the locked entrance so they know who is ringing the bell?

Always Practicing

So as martial artists, we're trying to train 24/7. Always practicing.

Always practicing what? Being in Condition Yellow, according to Jeff Cooper. If you do that, your whole world will change.

These systems come from people who have experienced what it takes and trained others to be ready in case something happens. To be present rather than in your own world and so self-absorbed you're oblivious to your surroundings, more caught up in not wanting to be interrupted from whatever it is you're doing even when the interruption may be life-threatening.

When you are in the moment and aware of your surroundings, your whole world changes. For one, you're not going to be caught up in what happened yesterday, what might be happening tomorrow. You certainly might think about it on occasion, but you're not caught up in it. You don't go there. You're Here. You're Now.

What Are Possible Ways We Can Practice This?

For one, when you enter a building you want to be aware. Think of the Ba Gua, "eight directions." From where you are, what do you see in the eight directions? Can you see the four walls and the corners of the room? What are your lines of sight to see what's going on in the room?

Your eyes should go to all eight directions, fully aware. Not paranoid, just take notice. Take notice and know where the exits are. If something goes down and it's all happening so fast, do you want to be trying to figure out where the exits are then? No.

If you make a habit to make a mental note where the exits are, then you already have it registered. You can even get in the habit of positioning yourself closer to an exit, or having a clear path, (though that may not always be practical). Now you know if something happens you will respond quicker and know immediately where to go. That's not stressful. That's preparation. And we can practice that all the time.

So, that's how we can walk down the street and practice awareness. How many cars passed by? What were their colors? Some people even talk about memorizing license plates, just for the fun of it, but taking notice of that kind of detail. Well, how many more ways can you practice awareness?

Go to a restaurant. Consider your position. You can't always control this but to the best of your ability, can you sit yourself where the wall is behind you, so then you can see the rest of the place? The best place to sit is where you have a line of sight to the entrance and to the exit, and you know exactly what to do if anything bad happens. You can see things. Things aren't blocked from your view, particularly the entrance because that's where the bad guy could come in.

If we're preparing for this active shooter scenario, we want to be able to see that entrance. If you see people freaking out at the entrance, you hit the exit as quickly as you can with your family or friend.

Okay, so I'm at my table, back to the wall or at least where I'm sitting I can see most of the room. Take notice. Is there a woman next to me or a man next to me? What kind of shoes are they wearing? How many people are behind the counter? Is it frantic? Are they very busy or are they kind of calm and going a little slower?

There are so many things you can notice like how many people are at the table next to me? What are they eating? When you leave the restaurant if you have kids you might test them by asking, "What was the person next to us wearing? Was it a man or a woman? How many people was she with? Were they calm? Were they having a good time or were they arguing?"

It's never too soon to create these habits. Then it becomes second nature.

People caught up in their own world, and all their troubles, don't notice these things at all. But what it does is it starts to open your mind to your surroundings. What color was the table? What did the placemat look like? Did it have some artwork on it or did it have some fun and games, or was there advertising? What kind of placemat? What did the menu look like? What color was the menu?

You can just make up things and keep finding out how much was noticed. Were there things on shelves up top? Was there art on the walls? What kind of art did you see? Did you notice the picture of the butterfly? Or what was the picture next to the one with the butterfly, on the left side? Was the frame light brown, dark brown, or black? Did it even have a frame?

Just play around with the possibilities, and you can test yourself, or again, if you're a parent you can test your children. You just get them used to playing this game, so everywhere they go they just start doing that. This kind of exercise will eventually open your mind to your surroundings on autopilot.

But like anything, it's difficult in the beginning. So you make it like a game, until it becomes something you do more and more unconsciously. That's not stressful. That's actually getting you more involved with your world, more open to your surroundings and into your world.

So again, Observe and Orient.

JANUARY 1, 2017 UPDATE: It is New Year's Day as I finish up here and prepare this book for the final stages to be edited, formatted, and published. And I am compelled to interrupt your reading as just this morning there was another nightclub attack, this time in Istanbul, Turkey. As reported in The Telegraph by Chris Graham and Nick Squires:

"A gunman reportedly dressed in a Santa costume killed at least 39 people, including 16 foreigners, at a famous nightclub in Istanbul during New Year's Eve celebrations.

Armed with a long-barreled weapon, the attacker shot a police officer before storming the elite Reina club in the Ortakoy area of the city at about 1.45am."

These attacks are not only continuing, they're becoming more frequent as well as more sinister. Really now, *dressed as Santa??*

By the time you are reading this, I wonder how many more attacks have occurred? How many more innocent civilians will die while out living their lives or having a good time oblivious to the imminent danger?

On a recent trip to Mexico, there were armed military guards all over the airport as well as throughout Mexico City. I also saw them many years ago, on the beach while vacationing in Acapulco. Is that what we want throughout the world?

The information here is just a start. Please, take it further and get informed, so you increase your odds of surviving if you happen to be caught in one of these life-threatening situations.

Back to the "Game" - Discovering Baseline

If I'm in a good position and I'm taking notice of my surroundings, and I'm playing this game, what do you think the most important thing I need to know is?

When we go on our retreat, we talk about having the opportunity to shift our minds to the natural world. There's a baseline in the natural world which is so much deeper and lower, calmer, more quiet and settled, than we have in our world.

Our world feels like constant chaos running around. In nature, it's very calm and quiet. And guess what happens when something changes that. One of the first things you'll notice is the quiet. The birds stop singing and all the rest of the wildlife goes still or hides.

Why do the birds go quiet? Something's up. They don't need to fly away because they're basically safe up there, but they're also going to be quieter if there's a predator. They can't fly away, the predator gets them. So all of a sudden, it's dead silence, something's up and you don't even see it but the birds do. That's my point.

Normally there is plenty of noise in the woods. But there isn't noise in the woods when you come in and disrupt things. So you may not have ever experienced what I'm talking about.

When we have our retreat every Fall, students are given plenty of opportunities to experience this for themselves. Of course, you can try it anytime if you can get to some woods. It may look and feel so desolate when you first arrive. However, if you sit quietly and don't move for 15 or 20 minutes, the natural world will come back to life because you were the initial threat. So you get to feel that baseline rhythm. What it's really like in their world.

Into Our World

So now you go to a restaurant, that's the question you must ask: "What is normal here? What's the baseline rhythm here?" If it's a busy place, you're going to see the workers moving around fast. There's going to be plenty of talking.

Then you might ask yourself, "What would not be normal here?"

For example, somebody sitting there looking uncomfortable. They may appear to be panicking, looking around with sweat coming down their face. What are they upset about? That might be something you pay attention to. You keep an eye on that person.

Are they upset because of their recent divorce or are they upset because they're wearing a bomb under their coat?

Two very different extremes but something doesn't fit. They're not acting according to what is considered normal in the current environment. Something's up, so keep an eye open.

Now the question is: "Should I do anything about it?"

It isn't enough to just take notice. You also have to take action when you recognize the anomaly. If nearby, you may ask, "Hey buddy, you okay?" Or, you may talk to security or the management to check it out. But you keep an eye on him to determine if further action is required. Should you run? Hide? Fight? Or do nothing?

Observation and orientation tell you what to do with that information.

You notice two people at a table, everybody's talking, and two people are very quiet. They don't say anything. You can take notice of that. That's not normal, but it may not be dangerous. They just don't talk. They don't get along, but it's different. There's something up with that relationship. You can take notice of that. Obviously, it's something different, not normal.

A library should be very quiet. Something loud in the library is really out of place. You might want to know what that is immediately. At a football game, you observe everybody yelling and making a lot of noise. That's normal. Everybody's yelling, screaming, making noise and rooting for their team. Somebody just sitting there, not paying attention to the game, might be a problem. That's not normal for the environment.

It's the anomalies. Something's different. And that's what you can just start practicing by taking notice. What's normal here, what's not normal here?

Something else you can look at is body language. There are dominance and submissiveness or one person being the bully. That shows aggression. That shows something that's out of the norm because most people want to get along.

The only way to start developing these skills is to be paying attention. You have to think about what's normal, what's not normal.

So find a good position so you can take in what's going on, establish a baseline of what's normal, and then practice, at least in your mind, what you could do if something happens.

For example, if a gunman walked through the entrance that is now across the room from where you are, what would you do? Do you go after the gunman? Do you run, hide or fight?

You should already know where the exits are. If the gunman is across the room, you run! You get out as fast as you can while screaming for everyone else to run too. You can shout two simple words: "GUN!" and "RUN!"

If you didn't at least get acquainted with the room enough to know where your exits are - especially what is nearest to where you are standing or sitting, you might go running across to where you came in because you freak out. There's the moment of "This isn't real" in your mind, and you just go for the first exit you can think of.

But if you planned ahead, and you should always plan ahead, then you can have a good time with your eyes always taking in the room. It can become just the way you live, aware of your surroundings. That's situational awareness.

What if you happen to be right where the gunman enters? What do you think? What might you do then? Would you do anything differently?

That's when you go after the gunman.

Think about it. If somebody did that in the Orlando nightclub maybe just a few people would have died. Maybe the person who jumped the gunman would have died, but they might have also saved 50 people.

Bravery is having the courage to do what must be done when it must be done. And there is no bravery without fear.

Unfortunately, most become the deer in headlights. This is the, "Oh my God I can't believe this is happening to me!" crowd. So, they just don't do anything. They freeze. They don't run away. They don't attack. They just freeze. And that's why they have no chance.

Let's work on not being one of those people.

If you practice what has been described here and if more people were taught to practice these things, we'd all be better able to thwart these attacks. There are excellent courses out there. Isn't your life and the lives of your loved ones worth the time and effort it takes to be better prepared?

It should be the norm that you know what to do, just like the many fire drills we've all been a part of. Everybody knows what to do because we practice that. Why not practice this?

The Fastest Wins

The most important thing about observe, orient, decide, and act is whoever does it fastest wins.

I must say that I can't imagine the lunatic gunman having any sort of skill or expectation whatsoever other than to aim and pull the trigger at a bunch of sitting ducks. So if you're a step ahead, you have a really good chance of taking him out. A really good chance. You might want to know how to disarm. That's the sort of thing we'll do at one of our retreats - how to disarm a weapon. You can find opportunities if you look.

It also helps to know how to attack and be able to hurt this person, so they're done. You don't want to be wrestling around with that gun going off and still killing people. So you've got to know how to disable, disarm, and put this guy out of commission quick.

Your awareness in the moment is what allows you to see what is happening and react before the person even realizes it. That person can be downed and hurt before they even realize what happened because they're human, too. They don't expect that. That's the last thing they expect - somebody fighting back.

That shooter in Orlando even had people shooting at him right at the beginning. He went in and was shooting people for three hours! People were trapped in restrooms or wherever they could hide just hoping and praying not to be found. That's a terrible thing. But nobody was able to just go after him. If even just a few people could rush him and smother him, they could have stopped it.

The thing is, few people have these tools. The average person doesn't have any idea what to do in this situation. In most cases, they also don't want to take the time to learn (last I heard only about 1-2% of people have martial arts training). Most just hope and pray the police can get there to help them. Apparently, in Orlando, they got there pretty quickly but... fifty people later.

No offense meant for law enforcement. Please don't misinterpret what I am writing here. It's simply logistics. They can't be everywhere all the time. And if there is any pre-conceived plan by the attacker, they already know things like: the civilians won't have guns, there is only one security guard, etc.

In most cases, the police can only write the report afterward. They can't be everywhere so we have to take responsibility and prepare to be ready just in case.

That's why it all starts with awareness.

We live in a world that has so many thousands of messages constantly coming at us. We even want to be distracted because life is hard, and so we want to enjoy our music and we want to be able to constantly be texting, posting on our Facebook, and whatever else we're doing. And then there's the constant multitasking. How often are you just doing what you're doing, actually just one thing? Not often for most. And that can quite literally get us killed.

Yeah, there's fifty out of how many, hundreds of millions. We may think the chances are extremely small. But those people never thought it would happen to them before that weekend. Did any of the people that it has happened to over these years think that it was going to happen to them? Sandy Hook, Columbine, Orlando, the Boston Marathon, the truck attacks in Nice, France or Berlin, Germany? Any other?

Did any of these people think that it could happen to them? Had anything in their lives up to that point prepared them for that fateful day?

That's the problem. It's such a surprise! Of course, as a martial artist, my thinking is everybody should learn martial arts. But everyone needs to learn martial arts in the way that I am describing where you're taught to train awareness all the time.

No Downtime. You Practice All the Time.

That doesn't mean punching or kicking or sitting in a horse stance 24/7. It means, as a martial artist you take life seriously. You always do what you can. Always learning. Always growing. Always aware and alert.

You do what you can to not get caught off guard. Can you still be caught off guard? Absolutely. I'm sure I can be caught off guard. But the more you practice, the less chance of that happening.

Then aware becomes the normal state. Always in Condition Yellow (never in Condition White!).

Condition White is where most people live.

Stalking Wolf, the teacher of the well-known and respected tracker and naturalist, Tom Brown Jr., would describe the average person's awareness akin to, "the land of the living dead," as they sleepwalk through their lives. They're just like robots or zombies walking around with no real connection to their world. The average person just goes about their business doing their thing and then when something unexpected happens they freeze.

I was fortunate enough to have taken a number of courses with Tom Brown, Jr. Because of what I learned from him, I found that in my experience the best place to work on my awareness is out in nature. I've spent a lot of time in the woods over the years. Just sitting quietly while expanding your awareness is a gateway to a whole new world.

And it's the quiet time that inspires courage.

A goal, then, is to always practice like you were there in the woods and opening your mind and all your senses. Then you'll more easily recognize when something is off. Don't ignore it.

As I said earlier, that's what changes lives. That's how this practice changes lives because you are more connected to your life. So now you're going to be less stressed and distracted or worried about the future. Because if you're more in the moment, you don't have time for that. You're not sitting there with your mind all over the place and worried about what might happen or what happened yesterday, and all the things you can't do anything about.

We spend so much mental energy and emotional energy on the things we can't do anything about from the past with guilt, and the future with worry and fear. The future is our imagination, and the past is our memories that can be completely off because it's just what you think happened, not necessarily what really happened.

So if you can practice getting out of your own way and getting through the programming, actually seeing the world as it is, not as we think it is but *as it really is*, and practice that all the time, your situational awareness will become more and more your natural state.

Go play those awareness games and enjoy getting good at it.

Isn't is always better to know what to do and never have to use that knowledge than be guessing when your life depends on it?

Conclusion

In conclusion, I hope this book has made it clear that there is so much more to martial arts than fighting.

Although I do believe in the importance and responsibility we each have of being able to protect ourselves or a loved one if it were ever necessary, most of the people I train stick around because of how their practice has positively impacted their everyday lives.

In addition to all the punching, blocking, kicking, and control techniques, it's the meditation and deeper philosophy - integral components of traditional martial arts - that changes lives.

In my experience, training both your body *and your mind* is the way to the highest levels of inner peace and happiness as well as mental, emotional, and physical health.

The martial artists of ancient times had to be focused. They had to be disciplined. They had to be in great physical shape.

Why?

Because their lives depended on it.

They were also highly respected. People knew what it took to develop those skills. They understood the dedication.

Today it makes sense to practice because of the reward of the practice itself. It makes our lives better. Our long-term students will be the first to tell you that.

If you've been training in any style of martial arts for any appreciable amount of time, I have one question: *"Is your life better because of it?"*

Are your relationships better? Is your job or career better? Are you more relaxed and better at handling stress? Are you better at letting go and playing when the time is right?

If you cannot answer, "Yes," then the next question must be, "Why not?" and, "What's missing in your training?"

I hope this book has helped answer that in some way.

Don't measure progress in your martial art training by the color around your waist. Measure only by how well it is positively impacting your life.

When you experience the concept of *achievement through consistent effort over time* - once again, the true meaning of *Kung Fu* - through your own invested "blood, sweat and tears" time into anything you pursue, you realize it's the only way to achieve anything of value in your life.

"The journey of a thousand miles begins with a single step." Lao Tzu

Traditional martial arts training is in harmony with moral, philosophical, and healing principles. Those who practice develop a higher sense of purpose and place in this world. They become more confident as well as optimistic.

This training changes lives.

You have an opportunity to become a part of this ancient tradition that simply makes more capable people with stronger minds and bodies *who believe in themselves.*

This practice was designed NOT for fighting but instead *to stop the fighting.*

Isn't that what you really want... to stop fighting every day - stop the mental, emotional, or physical confrontations - so you can have more peace, happiness, and fulfillment in your life?

And to work more *with* others in your life - at work, in relationships, at play - rather than against?

Learn to love the process of pursuing your goals. Kung Fu is a journey. Maybe you would like to enjoy the journey with us.

This training has been going on for thousands of years. Imagine yourself becoming a part of history.

If you are in the Bergenfield, NJ area and would like more information about our programs I encourage you to call us at 201-385-3130 to discuss your options. Or visit our website: www.BlueDragonKungFu.com.

If you are not in our area, please get in touch and let us know if you'd be interested in our distance learning program that is in the works.

You can also go to www.shifuahles.com/its-a-powerful-life and claim your FREE MEMBERSHIP where you'll have access to many inspirational talks, recorded live at our weekly meditation classes, going above and beyond the topics covered in this book.

Thank you for reading!

If you enjoyed this book I would be grateful if you would leave a brief honest review. To do that, please go to: bit.ly/amzn-powerful-review

Your positive review can really help other readers like you discover this book and hopefully enjoy it as much as you did.

Read what a few of our students have to say:

"**W**hat you said about what it means to you to be called Shifu is self-evident in your actions, your mannerism and the way you interact with your students. When I moved to Jerusalem I attended trial classes at eight different martial arts schools. What I found most lacking was an instructor who dedicated him/herself to the principles you talked about and who displayed a sense of responsibility toward their students as well as toward the teachings which they were passing down. It was a very difficult financial decision for me to re-enroll at your school but I believe a deciding factor is that you are someone that I can call Shifu. To me, to call you so is a sign of respect, trust, and acknowledgment that you represent, through your dedication to the traditions you are transmitting, an optimal lifestyle that I am trying to live up to. It means that you are someone I look up to on many different levels. It is rare to encounter people who are uncompromising when it comes to acting according to their values and the values and teachings you are passing on deeply resonate with me and the life I am trying to live. Nearly everyone in my life thinks trying to "be an ideal" is naive at best, and often destructive or worse. But I don't want to waste my life settling for what everyone else calls being realistic. I think you have created a space where people follow your initiative to reach into the depths of the universe and recognize those infinite possibilities as reality. It's an honor to be one of your students."

Elana Amminadav

"I was looking for a martial arts school that offered a balance of health and fitness, practical self defense, and appreciation for traditional philosophy. I found that and much more at this school. More than a place to train, this school is a community. Shifu Ahles and the senior instructors are such skilled, patient, generous and dedicated teachers I am inspired to strive and grow constantly. I found the other students, no matter how long they had been training, were also dedicated, welcoming and supportive. Anyone looking for a martial arts experience that is beyond kicking and punching, would do themselves a service to come visit Blue Dragon School of Martial Arts."

Leotis Sanders

"If you are looking to get in shape, have more confidence or learn how to defend yourself, you will find all that at the Blue Dragon School of Martial Arts. All of those things are a byproduct of the bodymind training that is the essence of this school. For me, the real value is learning a set of skills that can be applied to improve all aspects of life; health, work, school, relationships, you name it! Chief Instructor Shifu Ahles has provided an ideal place to learn true martial arts."

Frank Gallinagh

"This school is the real deal. It's what many other schools should be but aren't. I've been here for almost 10 years now (after practicing Tai Chi for many years, and Karate for several years). I thank my lucky stars I wandered in one day to try a class. This is a school that can (no lie) change your life. How? By being authentic, by being generous, by being truly wise about what it means to learn a martial art. It's taught me how to practice and how to persevere. It's taught me that there are no easy answers, no quick solutions, but if I train diligently and keep working on the insight I receive, I will be startled at the result. It also addresses what it means to be a martial artist - that becoming a martial artist involves the mind and spirit as well, that training the body with mental focus strengthens the bodymind connection. Most importantly, it's taught me that becoming a martial artist is not ultimately about learning to fight well (which you do anyway). It's about enriching my entire life - my work life, my personal relationships, and my role as a caring member of this world population. Finally, just a side note for anyone who does Tai Chi: I love Tai Chi (and still practice on occasion), but if you want to explore a whole other dimension in terms of Chi flow and development, give this school a shot. The Blue Dragon is a rare gem."

James Broaddus

"When you initially think 'martial arts' you immediately think of the physical side - how to learn to punch, kick, defend, attack, etc. You don't always necessarily think about your own body and what it needs. Before attending The Blue Dragon School of martial arts, I did a lot of research to find the right school for me. I wanted a place where not only I could learn how to defend, but to train my body properly. The Blue Dragon School exceeded my expectations and I'm continually surprised with what I learn. They are very patient, very kind, and really listen to your specific needs and help train YOU - and not just your body, your mind too, with meditation and breathing exercises which really help control your mind in ways I've never expected. The amount of dedication in the staff is inspiring as well as in the students. When you're there, you really want to do your best, and not because you want to show off, but something more - because you're really focusing on you and what you are able to accomplish within yourself. Martial Arts training took a whole new meaning for me once I started attending this school, and I'm very thankful to all the staff and my fellow peers. The longer I attend Blue Dragon, the more I look forward to coming to class each time and experiencing new things."

Theresa Finnelli

"The Blue Dragon School of Martial Arts is definitely a special place. It is one of the rare martial art schools that emphasizes a traditional approach to the study of kung fu. The traditional approach consists of training the body and mind through meditation and chi cultivation exercises. The style taught here is an intricate internal martial arts system called Pa Kua Chang (Ba Gua Zhang). It is unique because it is a style adaptable to any body type. In other styles, such as Karate or Tae Kwon Do you rarely see older practitioners performing the way they were when they were young. However, in Pa Kua Chang powerful movements are executed with fluidity by young and old practitioners which is one of the great aspects of our art."

Elena Karimova

"I have been with the school for almost 4 years. I tried numerous exercise programs including cycling, yoga, and various gyms and never stayed with any of them. After 6 months, I was bored to tears and found no improvement either physically or mentally. All of that changed when I joined Blue Dragon. After a few months, my body developed definition and muscle tone. My flexibility and strength improved. The Kung Fu classes give me a high intensity aerobics workout along with strength training. The Chi Kung classes improve my flexibility and endurance plus it provides a sense of calm that I had never experienced with either yoga or Tai Chi. I am 52 years old and I am in the best shape of my life. Shifu Ahles is a wonderful teacher and motivator. His energy and enthusiasm is contagious - so much so that my 10-year-old daughter, who also attends the school, absolutely loves it and hates to miss a class. It doesn't matter what age you are or your fitness level---Blue Dragon will change your life and on top of that, you will meet some amazing people. This is traditional kung fu and it is never boring. You'll constantly learn something new about kung fu and yourself."

Rose Mary Potter

"There would be a large void in my life without the Blue Dragon School of Martial Arts. I would miss the hard training, the expert tutelage of Shifu Ahles and the friendships that have been created with some of the other students. Attending class always has a positive effect on me no matter how tired I am or how difficult my day has been. Because of the training, I have become stronger, healthier and fitter. How can I argue with that? With the meditation and the hard training I have become more productive at work and perform at a much higher and calmer level. Also, my wife Jennifer has seen a positive change in my duties as a husband and a father."

Gerry Picardi

"I am so happy I found this school. I joined mainly to learn self defense, but had much self-doubt along the way, as I saw younger people learn so much quicker than I could. And it is still happening to this day, but it is the encouragement I get from everyone here and the feeling that no one is judging me but me, that keeps me going and trying to do my best, knowing that the results reflect the effort I put in. Being here is a great, constant lesson in accepting what is and being able to continue to live life to the best of my ability.

I joined for self defense so imagine my great surprise when I heard Shifu say that I will take my practice with me 24 hours a day. I could not imagine what he meant. Slowly but surely, this practice changed my life. I realized that it is not only the physical practice that strengthens you but also, the mental, spiritual practice. It is not only the punching and kicking but what you do with it, and how you use it - how to stop the fight. More importantly, this practice has helped me to stop the fight within me. Meditating has helped me to calm my mind and be able to think things through calmly.

The Lessons in Mindfulness* had a big impact on me. Some of the lessons helped me to really look at myself which was scary. I think that when you are young, the lessons have a different meaning than when you get to my age. For me, it was more a reflection of my life rather than what you want to achieve. It was sometimes difficult to truthfully answer all the questions, but again, it was part of this practice, it was a challenge that I overcame, and I am glad I did them. They are not written by Shifu, but they might as well have been.

As I age, I have noticed the difference in my strength and stamina, and also my mind. It takes me even longer to remember forms and techniques, but I accept that, and work to the best of my ability. I take everything as a personal challenge, and try not to give up. I am surrounded by a lot of negative people. Knowing that there are no coincidences, I wonder why? I now believe that this is one of my personal challenges, to not let these people bring me down, and to always appreciate what I have and where I am in life. They seem to like to talk to me because I just listen without judgment. Shifu's talks give me the strength to do this. I have realized that they don't really want to hear what I have to say, they just need someone to talk to, to get through whatever perceived crisis they are in.

I need to work more on my sparring but I do not like hitting people that I like. I need to look at my opponent directly. It makes a big difference in taking in the whole of what my opponent is presenting to me, the openings and their intentions. (And isn't that what I should be doing in life also?) I have to work on being smart as I know I am not as quick as the younger ones. I am aware that I should be realistic about my practice. Do I have a strong will or am I just stubborn? Is it time to just practice for exercise?

If I had not taken up this practice, I would have been struggling to understand my purpose in life after taking care of my family. Thanks to Shifu's talks and philosophy, I now know that I am here to be me, but the best me that I can be. Being here has also helped me to be a more confident person and be much more aware of my surroundings. The physical practice is a great challenge and motivation to keep going, the meditation keeps me sane and grounded. I feel like the practice is always with me and it is a good feeling."

Grace Chong

*Lessons in Mindfulness is a powerful two-year program created by Sifu Robert Brown that teaches the deeper philosophical aspects of the martial arts in a structured way.

One Last Thing!

Remember to go to
www.shifuahles.com/its-a-powerful-life
and claim your FREE GIFT!

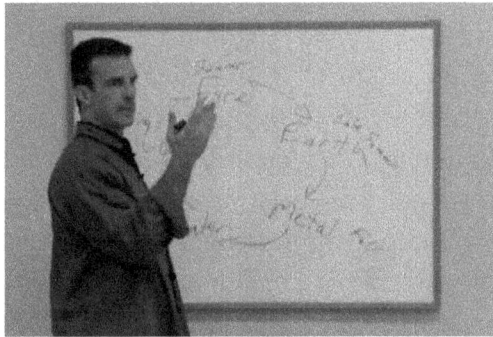

You have a FREE MEMBERSHIP waiting for you where you'll have access to many inspirational talks, recorded LIVE at our weekly meditation classes, that go above and beyond the topics covered in this book. If you liked this book, you'll love these talks!

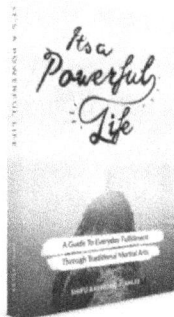

Acknowledgments

This book could not have been written without all the support of my wife, Nicolle, my parents, the great teachers, mentors, martial arts "brothers," and other amazing people who have influenced my thinking, contributed to my understanding of Natural Laws, inspired my passion for training and teaching traditional martial arts and to live A Powerful Life, (in chronological order):

Coach Greg Toal, the legendary high school football coach who made Don Bosco Prep a national powerhouse. In 1982 and 1983, at Saddle Brook High School, we were his first head coaching job, where he took a group of players who didn't win a game as freshmen to the state championship as seniors. Although we lost, it was an experience you never forget. I was fortunate enough to learn early on what a difference a great coach can make on the field and in life. Coach Toal's passion and work ethic was inspiring to experience. I'll never forget how he made us believe in ourselves, and to always strive for perfection in practice. He is, and always will be, a true winner and strong positive influence in my life. I'm still inspired by his frequent statement to each of us way back then, *"Do your job!"*

Gerry Lopez, who is mentioned in the beginning of this book. He inspired and influenced me early on, helping me to see things from a different perspective. Gerry got me started on my lifelong path of martial arts. He lives by what he learned through his Kung Fu training, and applies these life principles in his approach at his Hudson Square Salon in Hoboken, NJ. Truly, "good people," and still a great friend.

Master Randy Elia, my first teacher in the martial arts. I am grateful that he was there teaching traditional Kung Fu at a time when it was quite rare and hard to come by. He gave me my first opportunity to teach as his assistant. It was at his "Academy" that I fell in love with all the art had to offer, and decided my life path.

Dr. Yang Jwing-Ming, my second teacher, and who I owe so much to as he filled in the gaps of understanding that I was missing. On my many visits to Boston, he would sit me down next to him to meditate during our lunch breaks. He really took me under his wing and helped me to see behind the scenes in the world of Chinese martial arts in this country.

Grandmaster Park Bok-Nam, my Shifu for nearly 25 years, and to whom I owe my deepest gratitude for the martial arts education he provided. Through Shifu Park's teaching of the principles behind the arts, I have what I like to call a "litmus test" to be able to recognize quality, train effectively, and how to develop real skills. Thanks to him, I know how to create for myself, and not just copy what has been passed down, created by others. He truly taught me "how to fish" for myself.

Shifu Glen Moore, Grandmaster Park's most senior active student, and my "Big Brother." Shifu Moore has been instrumental in my learning process over all my years with Grandmaster Park. A lifetime martial artist and master in his own right, he has always been there for me through thick and thin. He is a true brother and friend.

Shifu Ion Ionescu, my training partner under Grandmaster Park for many years. Our weekly drives to Baltimore, (and wherever Shifu Park was for seminars) were always learning experiences and great conversations. We were inseparable at training camps, going off to train at every opportunity (since he always had endless energy!). It was with Shifu Ionescu that I learned how to create, (through hundreds of hours of frustration together!). Without him I don't think I would have gotten nearly as deep an understanding of the difficult style of Ba Gua Zhang, as taught by Grandmaster Park. He, too, is a true brother, friend, and the best training partner I could ever ask for.

Tom Brown Jr., and his student, Jon Young, where I was able to experience, first-hand, what I like to refer to as, "Practical Daoism," to become one with, and at home in, nature. Their knowledge of the natural world extends beyond the physical, and brings to life the teachings of the ancient sages and native peoples all over the world.

Sifu Robert Brown, my "brother from another mother," (or martial arts lineage) with whom I discovered ways to communicate and present my passion, and these great teachings, in a way that reaches more people, more deeply, than I ever could have figured out on my own. He is a true mentor to masters, and I am very grateful for the close relationship we have. If we get together, forget sleep, because we'll be up all night talking about martial arts.

I would also like to thank those who helped make this book a reality and to bring it to fruition: Thanks to Ida Fia Sveningsson, for cover design, the team at happyselfpublishing.com (including initial advice and editing by Phil Owens), Elana Amminadav for her valuable additional edits and style suggestions, and Bryan Cohen for his book description copywriting expertise. Also, as a recovering perfectionist, I must give special thanks to the writing/publishing step-by-step approach taught at Self Publishing School and their motto: "Done is better than perfect."

About the Author

Shifu Raymond J. Ahles, is a dedicated and dynamic teacher who is recognized by his students for both his skill and devotion to teaching. He emphasizes not just the physical aspects of martial arts training but the philosophy behind it. Knowing what a profound influence the martial arts can have on one's own personal development, he takes his responsibility to his students seriously and does everything possible to help them cultivate a greater sense of calm, focus and self-awareness, ultimately improving and enriching their everyday lives.

Shifu Ahles began his training in the Chinese martial arts in 1984 and has been actively teaching since 1986. He first studied with Master Randy Elia of Peter Kwok's Kung Fu Academy, where he completed all material available in the styles of Shaolin Chang Quan (Long Fist), Tai Ji Quan (Tai Chi), Ba Gua Zhang, Xing Yi Quan and Chin Na, the art of "seizing and controlling".

In 1988, he completed his Bachelor of Science Degree in Exercise Physiology with a concentration in Adult Fitness at Montclair State University. He is also an NSCA Certified Strength & Conditioning Specialist (CSCS) and a Certified Strongfirst Level 2 Kettlebell Instructor (SFG2).

He further enhanced his knowledge and understanding with well-known martial arts author and master Dr. Yang Jwing-Ming of Boston, Mass. Shifu Ahles studied privately with Dr. Yang and in regular classes at YMAA, Boston. With Dr. Yang, Shifu Ahles focused on the study of the Jian (Straight Double-Edge Sword) and Chin Na. He also trained in Shaolin Long Fist, Shaolin White Crane, White Crane Staff, and Tai Chi Push Hands.

Dr. Yang was instrumental in forming the perspective that Shifu Ahles has of the martial arts today and was a great early influence on his practice. From Dr. Yang, he learned the only way to become accomplished at anything was through patience, perseverance, and a strong will.

From 1991 to 2016, Shifu Ahles studied Ba Gua Zhang (Pa Kua Chang) under the personal instruction of Grandmaster Park Bok-Nam, with whom he was accepted as a 7th Generation "Lineage Disciple," and given the Chinese name, "Yi Fu," meaning "Firm Father (Teacher)." For nearly 25 years, he was an active student and member of the Ch'iang Shan Pa Kua Chang Association.

In 1992, he spent a short time in China to experience the culture and research the martial and healing arts with Dan Miller, the former editor of the now defunct, "Pa Kua Chang Journal" and writer of both volumes of Grandmaster Park's books, "The Fundamentals of Pa Kua Chang."

As a traditional progression from the martial arts to the healing arts, Shifu Ahles also has been professionally trained and certified in acupuncture and Chinese Medicine. While studying at the New York College for Wholistic Health and Medicine in Syosset, NY, he completed the Advanced Amma Therapy® (Chinese medical massage) program in 1997, and is a "Certified Amma Therapist" (C.A.T.); and the Oriental Medicine program (Traditional Chinese Medicine, including acupuncture and herbology) in 1998. He is National Board Certified in Oriental Medicine (Dipl.OM, NCCAOM) as well as a Licensed Acupuncturist (L.Ac.) and Chinese Herbalist in the State of New Jersey.

Shifu Ahles resides in northern New Jersey with his wife, Nicolle, and two amazing children, Forrest and Phoenix. He is the owner and Chief Instructor of the Blue Dragon School of Martial Arts in Bergenfield, where he continues to share his greatest passion.